Keto Diet for Women Over 50

The Ultimate Guide to Mastering Healthy Weight Loss with Ketogenic Lifestyle. Includes a 30-Day Meal Plan with Tasty Keto Recipes to Promote Longevity & Boost Your Energy

Dorothy Smith PhD

Table of Contents

Part One: Getting Started

Chapter 1: Keto Diet Explained

There are many diets gaining traction today, but none like the ketogenic diet. However, the interesting thing about this diet is that it is not used for weight loss. For the past century, it has been used as a way to treat epilepsy. However, because this diet is so temperamental, this is only done with the strictest doctor supervision. The ketogenic diet is a diet that is designed to release ketones in your bloodstream. Many of the cells in your body prefer to use blood sugar, which it gets from carbohydrates, as your body's main source of energy. The idea of the ketogenic diet is to put your body in a state of ketosis. This means the absence of circulating blood sugar from food and your body breaking down stored fat into the molecules called ketone bodies. When you reach ketosis, it is believed that more of your cells will use the ketone bodies for generating energy until you eat carbs again. This varies between person to person, so you need to be careful.

A warning that this book will give you before we proceed is that the ketogenic diet is not considered to be safe. Doctors all over the world and from the most prestigious medical practices advise against it for a few reasons. The first being that this diet was only invented to help people in the most extreme situations and even then not forever. Doctors recommend this diet for no longer than six months and even then only under constant contact and supervision by a doctor that you see. It has also been shown to put certain people into a state called ketoacidosis, which can be fatal. This is especially true in diabetics. They could die in under an hour. It can also worsen those with kidney disease as well as making you have sleep problems and stomach issues along with constipation and vomiting. Another downside is this diet has been shown to be heavy on red meat and other processed foods that are salty and fatty, which is unhealthy. You should also avoid keto if your pregnant as it could harm your unborn child as well as yourself.

That being said, the ketogenic diet is a diet that lacks carbohydrates and concentrates on proteins and fats. There are four different types of ketogenic diets, and you should be aware of all four as they differ in certain aspects. The first diet is the targeted diet. This will allow you to eat carbs, but you can only do so around workouts.

The next is the high protein diet. This one is similar to the basic diet, but obviously, it will include more protein. The numbers that this diet offers is 5% carbs, 35% protein, and 60% fat.

The third is the cyclical diet. This diet involves what is known as refeeding. The basis for this diet is that you have periods of higher-carb refeeds. For example, you have five ketogenic diet days and then two high carb days.

The last diet is the basic diet. This is the one that is used most often and by most people. The numbers for this one are as follows, 75% fat with only 5% carbs and 20% protein.

It is worth noting that the only two diets that have been studied extensively are the basic and high protein diet. The other two are more advanced, and bodybuilders and athletes are the ones that generally use them, although it's not ideal or recommended since they need further study.

The ketogenic diet believes that it is an effective way to lose weight and help lower your risk factors for disease.

It is also believed to be filling, and you can lose weight without having to count your calories or track what you're eating. However, this isn't true. The ketogenic diet makes you track your food very carefully because you need to know where your fat and carbs are, as well as the protein content. If you're not tracking these things, you could throw yourself out of where you are supposed to be.

Another benefit is that it is believed that it can help with diabetes. This is because it can help you lose excess fat, which is very closely related to diabetes. Especially type 2 diabetes. One study found that it can improve insulin sensitivity by 75%. However, this should be looked into more as other studies have found problems with this diet. Another belief is that it can help with cancer, Alzheimer's disease, and heart disease.

We have already mentioned that it has been used to treat epilepsy, but it is also said that it can help with polycystic ovary syndrome or PCS for short as well as Parkinson's disease. Brain injuries have been studied in one animal study, but there is much more research that is needed to be conclusive. On the lower scale, it may be able to help with acne as well.

Why is the keto diet so effective for weight loss? If you don't consume enough carbs from your food; your cells will begin to burn fat for the necessary energy instead. Your body will switch over to ketosis for its energy source as you cut back on carbs and calories.

Two elements that occur when your body doesn't need the glucose:

The Stage of Lipogenesis: If there is a sufficient supply of glycogen in your liver and muscles, any excess is converted to fat and stored.

The Stage of Glycogenesis: The excess of glucose converts to glycogen and is stored in the muscles and liver. Research indicates that only about half of your energy used daily can be saved as glycogen.

Your body will have no more food (similar to when you are sleeping) making your body burn the fat to create ketones. Once the ketones break down the fats, which generate fatty acids, they will burn-off in the liver through beta-oxidation. Thus, when you no longer have a supply of glycogen or glucose, ketosis begins and will use the consumed/stored fat as energy.

The keto diet will set up your body to deplete the stored glucose. Once that is accomplished, your body will focus on diminishing the stored fat you have saved as fuel. Many people don't understand that counting calories don't matter at this point since it is just used as a baseline. Your body doesn't need glucose which will trigger these two stages:

The State of Glycogenesis: The excess of glucose converts itself into glycogen which is stored in the muscles and liver. Research indicates only about <u>half</u> of your energy used daily can be saved as glycogen.

The State of Lipogenesis: This phase is introduced when there is an adequate supply of glycogen in your liver and muscles, with any excess being converted to fat and stored.

Your body will have no more food (similar to the times when you are sleeping) making your body burn the fat to create ketones. Once the ketones break down the fats, which generate fatty acids, they will burn-off in the liver through beta-oxidation. Thus, when you no longer have a supply of glycogen or glucose, ketosis begins and will use the consumed/stored fat as energy.

When the glycerol and fatty acid molecules are released, the ketogenesis process begins, and acetoacetate is produced. The Acetoacetate is converted to two types of ketone units:

Acetone: This is mostly excreted as waste but can also be metabolized into glucose. This is the reason individuals on a ketogenic diet will experience a distinctive smelly breath.

Beta-hydroxybutyrate or BHB: Your muscles will convert the acetoacetate into BHB which will fuel your brain after you have been on the keto diet for a short time.

There are many foods that you can eat on this diet, but there are many foods that you can't, and its this subject, in particular, that we're going to go into now. The following foods that you need to avoid eating are the following.

- Fruit- You will need to avoid all fruits except small portions of certain kinds like berries.
- Beans- Peas and beans like kidney beans are to be avoided as well because they are too high in carbs.
- Legumes- Lentils will also need to be avoided.
- Starches and grains -Wheat products like pasta and cereal are a big no-no, and you will have to stay away from these as well.
- Sugary foods- fruit juice, smoothies, junk food, and things like ice cream and cake are out as well.
- sugar -free foods-These are most often found in sugar alcohols or diet foods that claim to help you lose weight. They are very highly processed, and they can affect your ketone levels in a negative way.
- Alcohol-The carb content on these is very high, and they can knock you out of where you need to be.
- Root vegetables or tubers-This category means potatoes (including sweet potatoes) and things like carrots.

- Unhealthy fats-You should seriously limit your intake of the fats that are processed. This includes mayonnaise and vegetable oil.
- Diet items and low-fat items-These are overloaded with carbs and are extremely processed.
- Condiments and sauces- They contain too much sugar and fat that is unhealthy.

The foods that you should eat on this diet to make sure that you are following it correctly are the following. As we have stated above, some of these foods are unhealthy such as forms of coconut oil and red meats.

- Healthy oils-The three main ones to focus on are avocado oil, extra virgin olive oil, and coconut oil.
- Cheese-You can eat many different varieties, such as mozzarella, cheddar, cream, or blue. You should go for unprocessed cheeses.
- Eggs-Look for omega-3 whole eggs or pastured eggs.
- Fatty fish-Salmon, tuna, mackerel, and trout are all good options for you.

- Meat-Turkey, bacon, chicken, and sausage are all good options. Red meat and steak are other options as well.
- Butter-Try and get grass-fed if you can.
- Cream- As with butter, if you can find grass-fed, then go for that.
- Nuts-Almonds and walnuts are great options here.
- Seeds-Pumpkin seeds, flax seeds, and chia seeds are all good options, but a warning is that many seeds can cause issues with your digestion and stomach.
- Low carb vegetables-Most green vegetables are alright, and you can have peppers, onions, and tomatoes as well.
- Avocados-You can use them for guacamole, or you can eat them whole. Whole avocados can be used for so many recipes.
- Spices-You can use herbs and spices (healthy ones) and salt and pepper in moderation, of course.

Other healthy foods that you can eat as long as you are careful because the numbers vary as far as carbs (though most are zero and others go as high as 7 grams).

- Lamb
- Jerky
- Veal
- Bison
- Venison
- Sardines
- Shellfish (careful on this one the carbs will add up)
- Catfish
- Cod
- Herring
- Lobster
- Haddock
- Broccoli
- Cauliflower
- Brussels sprouts
- Kale
- Eggplant
- Asparagus
- Cucumber
- Mushrooms
- Green beans

- Celery
- Spinach
- Cabbage
- Swiss chard
- Zucchini
- Olives
- Strawberries
- Grapefruit (be careful on this one the carbs can get really high very quickly)
- Apricots
- Lemons
- Kiwis
- Mulberries
- Oranges
- Raspberries
- Peanuts
- Sunflower seeds
- Pistachios
- Macadamia nuts
- Hazelnuts
- Cashews
- Coconuts
- Full fat yogurt
- Greek yogurt
- Lard

- Tallow
- Coffee
- Tea
- Carbonated water
- Club soda
- Dark chocolate (choose a real dark chocolate with 70 percent cocoa at least)

Food is such an important part of this diet that it's important to make sure that you're informed on it so that you can have the best knowledge and the knowledge that is going to be of the most useful to you. Having the right information means you can be successful; having the wrong information can lead to injuries or worse. Doctors have said that you should always ask them before starting this diet at all, but this is proven to be more true if you have the following health issues.

- Obesity
- Heart conditions
- High blood pressure
- Diabetes
- Kidney issues
- Cancer

- Epilepsy

The reason that you should have their supervision is because these are all serious conditions. Especially things like cancer and epilepsy.

Exercise is so important on this diet as well, and it is important to understand how you need to utilize it for your benefit. Exercise is important in any diet that you choose, and it's important to be able to understand that exercise is what you need to become a healthier person, but it can actually be harder on the keto diet because your body is being put through so much already.

As such, your routine is going to change. The main reason is because your not using carbs for energy and fuel, your using fat for fuel. Fat doesn't give you that energy burst that you need for push-ups or jumps like carbs do. You will probably not feel like working out at all because of how your feelings, but you will be able to get past this, and you will be able to make a good routine for yourself.

Because workouts like sprinting, weightlifting, and high-intensity interval training are workouts all require that quick burst of energy, they are going to be much more strenuous though many say it won't be impossible. Just remember the reason for this is because the fat in your body is not as available to your muscles as the energy that you get from carbs are. Because of this, you are more likely to get tired during these workouts and much quicker than you usually do.

This doesn't mean you have to stop working out; it means you have to be smarter about how you work out. Jogging and bike riding are both great options for you to do on this diet, and a good rule of thumb is to go for something that is low to moderate as far as your workout and do something for a short duration. This is especially true for the first two weeks that you start this. With your doctor's permission, you can talk to them about going into higher amounts of workout, but you need to have their help with this, so check with them first.

If your feeling drained on the basic diet, another option is to try the targeted diet or the cyclical diet. This is not recommended for a lot of people, so this would be another area where you need to check with your doctor as well to see if this is alright for you. Another issue with doing this is that you will knock yourself out of that ketosis state that they want you to stay in. Overall, it has been proven that working out doesn't feel as good on the keto diet as it did before. This is another reason that the keto diet isn't for everyone. If you love exercising, this isn't the best choice for you. This is especially true because exercise is important for health.

It is recommended that along with speaking to your doctor about what exercises are good for you to do for yourself, is to speak to a nutritionist professional and a certified trainer as well. This will make sure that you have a great workout plan that is safe. You should also not do any workouts that you haven't done before. This is because this diet can affect how that workout is going to affect you, and the result could be very negative. Other tips that you need to be aware of is that when your working out on this diet are the following tips.

Listen to your body and what it's telling you. You should never keep going or pushing if your body is telling you it can't do it or handle it. If your body is telling you to stop, then you need to stop. Feelings of dizziness and exhaustion or even just fatigue are all signs that you should stop. They are not normal, and this is a sign that your body isn't responding well to this diet and that you need a doctor's help.

Make sure that you are eating enough. This is another big thing with this diet, and this doesn't just include keeping your calorie count where it needs to be. This means keeping your fat where it needs to be, as well. Remember that when your exercising, your body normally uses carbs then fat. Now your using fat. So if you're not taking in enough nutrition, you are not going to be able to handle even the simplest workout. You could actually be putting yourself in danger.

Avoid high-intensity workouts. This is so important with the keto diet. More is not better. In many cases, this is something that is true. The keto diet is considered to be an extreme diet, and as such, you won't be able to do what you are normally able to do. You have to be able to understand that high-intensity workouts are something that is no longer going to be able for you to do. Instead, remember that you really need to stick to a lower intensity workout instead. This is really important particularly important when your starting this diet and for at least the first month that you're doing this.

This diet puts a lot of stress on your body, and it can take a very long time to adjust if your actually able to adjust at all. Many people can't, and this is something to be aware of when you try. Don't push yourself too hard on this diet, or you will end up hurting yourself. If you pace yourself and eat well, you may be able to adjust and lose weight.

Some ideas for working out when you're doing the keto diet that are lower intensity are the following.

- Rowing
- Hiking

Gymnastics is also good for preventing injury and improving flexibility as well as improving how you move.

An example of a low-intensity workout that you can do is walking. This is easy to do, and it is great for losing weight. Swimming is another good activity though it straddles the fence. If you go lightly and keep it in the low-intensity area, then you are alright. If you push too hard it could be dangerous. When you are able to keep this thought in mind you will be able to perform exercises safely and make sure that they are working for you, not against you.

Chapter 2: Tips for Success

Routines are very important on this diet, and it's something that will help you stay healthy. As such, in this chapter, we are going to be giving you tips and tricks to make this diet work better for you and help you get an idea of routines that you can put in place for yourself.

Tip number one that is so important is DRINK WATER! This is absolutely vital for any diet that your on, and you need it if not on one as well. However, this vital tip is crucial on a keto diet because when you are eating fewer carbs, you are storing less water, meaning that you are going to get dehydrated very easily. You should aim for more than the daily amount of water however, remember that drinking too much water can be fatal as your kidneys can only handle so much as once. While this has mostly happened to soldiers in the military, it does happen to dieters as well, so it is something to be aware of.

Along with that same tip is to keep your electrolytes. You have three major electrolytes in your body. When you are on a keto diet, your body is reducing the amount of water that you store. It can be flushing out the electrolytes that your body needs as well, and this can make you sick. Some of the ways that you can fight this is by either salting your food or drinking bone broth. You can also eat pickled vegetables.

Eat when your hungry instead of snacking or eating constantly. This is also going to help, and when you focus on natural foods and health foods, this will help you even more. Eating processed foods is the worst thing you can do for fighting cravings, so you should really get into the routine of trying to eat whole foods instead.

Another routine that you can get into is setting a note somewhere that you can see it that will remind you of why you're doing this in the first place and why it's important to you. Dieting is hard, and you will have moments of weakness where you're wondering why you are doing this. Having a reminder will help you feel better, and it can really help with your perspective.

Tracking progress is something that straddles the fence. A Lot of people say that this helps a lot of people and you can celebrate your wins, however, as everyone is different and they have different goals, progress can be slower in some than others. This can cause others to be frustrated and sad, as well as wanting to give up. One of the most important things to remember is that while progress takes time, and you shouldn't get discouraged if you don't see results right away. With most diets, it takes at least a month to see any results. So don't get discouraged and keep trying if your body is saying that you can. If you can't, then you will need to talk to your doctor and see if something else is for you.

You should make it a daily routine to try and lower your stress. Stress will not allow you to get into ketosis, which is that state that keto wants to put you in. The reason for this being that stress increases the hormone known as cortisol in your blood, and it will prevent your body from being able to burn fats for energy. This is because your body has too much sugar in your blood. If you're going through a really high period of stress right now in your life, then this diet is not a great idea. Some great ideas for this would be getting into the habit or routine of taking the time to do something relaxing, such as walking and making sure that you're getting enough sleep, leads to the next routine that you need to do.

You need to get enough sleep. This is so important not just for your diet but also for your mind and body as well. Poor sleep also raises those stress hormones that can cause issues for you, so you need to get into the routine of getting seven hours of sleep at night on the minimum and nine hours if you can. If you're getting less than this, you need to change the routine you have in place right now and make sure that you establish a new routine where you are getting more sleep. As a result, your health and diet will be better.

Another routine that you need to get into is to give up diet soda and sugar substitutes. This is going to help you with your diet as well because diet soda can actually increase your sugar levels to a bad amount, and most diet sodas contain aspartame. This can be a carcinogen, so it's actually quite dangerous. Another downside is that using these sugar substitutes just makes you want more sugar later. Instead, you need to get into the habit of drinking water or sparkling water if you like the carbonation.

Staying consistent is another routine that you need to get yourself into. No matter what you are choosing to do, make sure it's something that you can actually do. Try a routine for a couple of weeks and make serious notes of mental and physical problems that you're going through as well as any emotional issues that come your way. Make changes as necessary until you find something that works well for you and that you can stick to. Remember that you need to give yourself time to get used to this and time to get used to changes before you give up on them.

Be honest with yourself, as well. This is another big tip for this diet. If you're not honest with yourself, this isn't going to work. Another reason that you need to be honest with yourself is if something isn't working you need to be able to understand that and change it. Are you giving yourself enough time to make changes? Are you pushing too hard? If so, you need to understand what is going on with yourself and how you need to deal with the changes that you're going through. Remember not to get upset or frustrated. This diet takes time, and you need to be able to be a little more patient to make this work effectively.

Getting into the routine of cooking for yourself is also going to help you so much on this diet. Eating out is fun, but honestly, on this diet, it can be hard to eat out. It is possible to do so with a little bit of special ordering and creativity, but you can avoid all the trouble by simply cooking for yourself. It saves time, and it saves a lot of cash.

This next topic falls into both the tip and routine category. Get into the habit of cleaning your kitchen. It's very hard to stick to a diet if your kitchen is dirty and full of junk food. Clear out the junk (donate it if you can, even though it's junk, there are tons of hungry people that would appreciate it) and replace all of the bad food with healthy keto food instead. Many people grab the carbs like crazy because they haven't cleared out their cabinets, and it's everywhere they look. Remember, with this diet, no soda, pasta, bread, candy, and things of that nature. Replacing your food with healthy food and making a regular routine of cleaning your kitchen and keeping the bad food out is going to help you be more successful with your diet, which is what you want here.

Getting into the routine of having snacks on hand is a good idea as well. This keeps you from giving into temptation while your out, and you can avoid reaching for that junk food. You can make sure that they are healthy, and you will be sticking to your high-intensity diet, which is what you want. There are many different keto snacks that you can use for yourself and to eat. We will have a list of recipes in the following chapters to help this as well.

A good tip would be to use keto sticks or a glucose meter. This will give you feedback on whether your users do this diet right. The best option here is a glucose meter. It's expensive, but it's the most accurate. Be aware that if you use ketostix, they are cheaper, but the downside is that they are not accurate enough to help you. A perfect example is that they have a habit of telling people their ketone count is low when they are actually the opposite.

Try not to overeat as this will throw you out of where you need to be. Get into the routine of paying attention to what your eating and how much. If this is something that you're struggling with, try investing in a food scale. You will be able to see exactly what it is your eating and make sure that your understanding your portions and making sure you stay in ketosis.

Another tip is to make sure that you're improving your gut health. This is so important. Your gut is pretty much linked to every other system in your body, so make sure that this something that you want to take seriously. When you have healthy gut flora, your body's hormones, along with your insulin sensitivity and metabolic flexibility will all be more efficient. When your flexibility is functioning at an optimal level, your body is able to adapt to your diet easier. If it's not, then it will convert the fat your trying to use for energy into body fat.

Batch cooking or meal prepping is another routine that is a good thing to get into. This is an especially good routine for on the go women. When you cook in batches, you are able to make sure that you have meals that are ready to go, and you don't have to cook every single day, and you can save a lot of time as well. You will also be making your environment better for your diet because you're supporting your goals instead of working against them.

The last tip is to mention exercise again. Getting into the routine of exercising can boost your ketone levels, and it can help you with your issues on transitioning to keto. Exercises also use different types of energy for your fuel that you need. When your body gets rid of the glycogen storages, it needs other forms of energy, and it will turn into that energy that you need. Just remember to avoid exercises that are going to hurt you. Stay in the smaller exercises and lower intensity.

Following these tips and getting into these routines is going to help you stay on track and make sure that your diet will go as smoothly as it possibly can.

Part Two: 30 Day Meal Plan

Are you a busy mom that's on the go? Or maybe you work in an office, and you only get a small amount of time to eat? Whatever your situation is, we've got recipes that are easy to make and just as easy to take with you, so you don't have to worry about missing a meal or not having enough time to eat. Some of the recipes that we will be showing you in the following chapters can be done in as few as ten minutes! It doesn't get any easier than that.

We will show you breakfast recipes first and then go in order of the meals with snacks at the end. So let's get started! A side note for all of the recipes is that only you know what you need in terms of carbs, calories, fat, and so on. As such, you are free to mix and match based on your personal needs. As a special note, these recipes have nutritional information, and they are based on serving.

Chapter 3: Breakfast Recipes

Avocado and eggs

Time needed to prepare: 20 minutes

This will give you a single serving

What you need:

- 3 free-range eggs (use large)
- 3 thin slices of bacon (cut them into small pieces)
- A single tablespoon of butter (use salted)
- A single avocado (remove the stone and cut the avocado in half)

What you need to do:

1. Scoop out your flesh of avocado. Be sure to leave a half-inch around the avocado.
2. Put a saucepan on a heat that is low before adding in your butter.
3. While it's melting, crack your eggs and beat them.
4. Add your bacon to the pan and let them dry on their own for a few minutes before adding your eggs to the opposite side of your pan.
5. Stir frequently during your scrambling.
6. The bacon and eggs should both be finished five minutes after you have added the eggs to the pan.

7. If you have finished the eggs, first take them out before finishing the bacon.
8. Mix the bacon pieces and your eggs before adding them to the avocado halves.

Nutritional information:

- Calories-500
- Fiber-8 grams
- Protein-25 grams
- Carbs-11 grams
- Fat-40 grams

Lemon smoothie

You will need 5 minutes for this

You will get 4 servings for this

You will need:

- A third of a cup of lemon juice (freshly squeezed)
- A quarter of a cup of powdered Swerve Sweetener
- A third of a cup of water
- 2 cups of ice
- A cup of yogurt (Greek)
- A cup of raspberries (frozen)
- 2 ounces of cream cheese
- A single teaspoon zest from a lemon

What you need to do:

- Get a blender.
- Add all of your ingredients.
- Blend until its a smooth consistency.

Nutritional information:

- Calories-148
- Fat-9.67 grams
- Fiber-1.06 grams
- Protein-5.41 grams
- Carbs-8.48 grams

Egg casserole

Time needed to prepare: 50 minutes

- The reason that this is on the list for women on the go is that you can make this the night before or early in the morning and it will give you eight servings which means that you can take servings with you and have leftovers and not have any cooking prep for other days.

This will give you eight servings

What you need:

- Half a dozen bacon slices (six)
- A dozen eggs (12 and use large)
- 10 ounces cheddar cheese (use shredded)
- 4 ounces of sour cream
- Cooking spray (use avocado oil spray)
- 4 ounces heavy whipping cream
- ⅓ of a cup of chopped green onions (this is optional but adds some great flavor to the dish)

What you need to do:

Preheat your oven to 350 degrees.
1. Cook your bacon on the stove before crumbling into bite-sized pieces after it has cooled, so you don't burn yourself.
2. Crack your eggs in a bowl before adding the cream.

3. Mix in a blender until it has combined well.
4. Spray a casserole pan with the spray before placing the cheese in a layer before adding the egg mix and bacon over the top.
5. Bake for thirty-five minutes.
6. Check it after a half-hour.
7. Remove from the oven when the edges have turned a color that looks golden brown.
8. Cool before cutting and placing your onions on top.

Nutritional Information:

- Calories-437
- Protein-43 grams
- Carbs-2 grams
- Fat-38 grams

As far as breakfast goes, this is a good one. You get a huge protein-packed breakfast, and it's got that fat you want as well. Just remember to be aware of your numbers. If you eat this much protein, now be careful to make sure that you're not going over later.

Broccoli Bread

This will take 35 minutes in total to prepare

It will give you ten servings

What you will need:

- A single cup of cheddar cheese (make sure that it is shredded)
- 5 eggs (make sure that they are beaten)
- 3 ½ tablespoons of flour (you should use coconut)
- 2 tsp of baking powder
- ¾ of a cup of broccoli florets (you need to make sure that they are raw, fresh, and chopped)

What you need to do:

1. Heat your oven to 350.
2. Spray a pan with cooking spray.
3. Mix all of your ingredients in a bowl before pouring it in the pan.
4. Bake for half an hour.
5. Add five minutes if necessary. It should be golden and puffed.
6. Slice into servings.

If you want to reheat this, all you have to do is use the microwave.

Nutritional information:

- Calories-90
- Fat-6 grams
- Protein- 6 grams
- Carbs- 2 grams
- Fiber-1 gram

Pizza

Time you will need: 25 minutes

You will be able to get two servings from this

What you will need:

- 4 eggs
- 2 cups of cauliflower (make sure that it is grated)
- 2 tablespoons of flour (make sure it's coconut)
- A single tablespoon of husk powder (use psyllium and make sure it's a brand that is mold-free)
- Olive oil, avocado, spinach, spices and herbs, and salmon (smoked) for toppings for the pizza to offer flavor and nutrients

What you need to do:

1. Heat your oven to 350 before lining a pizza tray with parchment.
2. Add all of the ingredients except what you will be using for the top of the pizza and mix into a bowl.
3. Set it aside.
4. Let it sit for at least five minutes, so the husk and flour are able to absorb the liquid that they need to.
5. Pour the base of the pizza in the pan. Go slow and be careful before molding it into a round pizza crust and make sure that it is even.

6. Let it bake for a quarter of an hour (fifteen minutes).
7. It should be fully cooked and golden brown.
8. Remove and top with your chosen items.

Nutritional information:

- Calories -454
- Fat-31 grams
- Carbs- 26 grams
- Protein-22 grams
- Fiber-17.2 grams

Pizza for breakfast? Yes, please! Now you will see that the carbs for this breakfast is a little high. This is why you can play with what you put on the pizza to create less carbs if you like.

Donuts

Time you will need for this: 40 minutes

You will be able to get 6 servings with this

What you will need:

- 2 eggs (make sure they are large)
- A single cup of flour (almond and blanched)
- A single tablespoon of cinnamon
- ½ of a teaspoon of vanilla extract
- 2 teaspoons of baking powder (use gluten-free)
- ⅓ of a cup of erythritol
- ¼ of a cup of butter (this will need to be solid when you measure, then melted and it needs to be unsalted as well)
- ¼ of a cup of milk (it needs to be almond and unsweetened)

For the coating for the donuts:

- 3 tablespoons of butter (same steps as above. Measure it solid, melt it and then make sure that you have chosen a butter that is unsalted)
- 1 teaspoon of cinnamon
- ½ of a cup of erythritol

What you need to do:

1. Heat your oven to 350 before greasing a donut pan and greasing it well.

2. Mix your ingredients (the dry ones) in a bowl.
3. In a separate bowl, mix in your eggs, milk, butter, and vanilla extract.
4. Mix the wet bowl into the dry bowl.
5. When you have made the batter, transfer it into the donut spots in the donut pan. Don't fill them all the way. Fill it a little more than half.
6. Bake for 25 minutes. If you have a silicone pan, you will have to go longer.
7. When it is done, they should be a nice and even golden brown color.
8. Let cool.
9. Remove from pan.
10. In a bowl, mix the dry ingredients for the topping.
11. When the donuts are cool, remove them from the mold and brush the side of the donut with the butter before pressing the mix of dry ingredients on top. It should create a crust.
12. Repeat for the other five donuts before eating.

Nutritional information:

- Calories-257
- Fat-25 grams
- Protein-6 grams
- Fiber-2 grams
- Carbs-5 grams

Crepes

You will need 15 minutes for this

You will be able to get 2 from this

What you will need:

- A single tablespoon husk powder (use a psyllium version)
- A single tablespoon of sweetener (if you are sticking to the tip that we have told you above you can cut this part out)
- ⅓ of a cup of water (make sure it's boiling)
- 3 eggs
- 3 tablespoons of flour (use coconut)

For the filling of the crepes:

- ½ of a cup of berries (raspberries or strawberries)
- A single ounce of dark chocolate (use the tip we gave you in the previous chapters)
- ½ of a tablespoon of oil or butter (if you are using oil use coconut)

What you need to do:

1. Mix the flour, husk, sweetener if you are going to use it, and the eggs into a boil.
2. Mix in your water and make sure it combines well.

3. In a pan that is nonstick, add in a single tablespoon of oil and turn up the heat to a medium level.
4. Add in no more than half of the liquid for the crepes and allow them to cook until the edges have turned brown.
5. Flip it over.
6. Cook until golden brown.
7. This should take no more than five minutes per crepe.
8. Repeat until all the dough is finished.
9. If you have chosen to add berries and chocolate, then you will need to melt your chocolate first before adding a spoonful to the middle of the crepe and adding the berries.
10. Close it up.
11. If you choose top with additional chocolate or berries for extra flavor.

Nutritional information:

- Calories-167
- Carbs-5 grams
- Protein-7 grams
- Fat-12 grams
- Fiber-5 grams

Omelette

You will need 17 minutes for this

You will get 2 servings for this

What you need:

- 7 ounces of spinach (frozen)
- Half of a dozen large eggs (six)
- 2 tablespoons of milk (you should use heavy cream or almond milk)
- 2 teaspoons of oil for frying (we are going to use olive oil)
- A single tablespoon of herbs (chives or parsley is good, but you need to make sure that they are fresh)
- A quarter of a cup of grated sharp cheddar
- A quarter of a cup of grated parmesan cheese
- A quarter of a cup of crumbled, mild feta cheese
- A single handful of kale that is chopped (discard the stems)
- A half of a cup of ricotta cheese
- Pepper for taste

What you will need to do:

1. Make sure that there is no liquid in your spinach. If there is, then you will need to squeeze it out. You should have a small handful left.
2. Chop the spinach finely then do the same with the kale (a food processor makes this easier and quicker).

3. Add the parmesan cheese along with cheddar, eggs, and milk and mix it well so it will combine well.
4. Mix the herbs, feta, and ricotta in a separate bowl and then season with pepper.
5. Place the bowl to the side.
6. Heat a single teaspoon of olive oil in a pan that is non-stick.
7. Pour in half of the egg mix you made.
8. On medium-high heat fry until just set.
9. Add half of the ricotta mix on top before folding the omelette over.
10. Be careful when you do this.
11. Place a lid over the pan and then cook for another minute so that your filling is warmed.
12. Repeat for the second omelette.

Nutritional information:

- Calories-522
- Fat-34.7 grams
- Fiber-2.4 grams
- Protein-44 grams
- Carbs-10.3 grams

Cheesy Bread

You will need 30 minutes for this

You will get 8 servings from this

You will need:

- A single egg
- A single tablespoon of cream cheese
- ¾ of a cup of mozzarella cheese
- A single teaspoon of basil
- A single tablespoon of garlic powder.
- 2 tablespoons of flour (you should use almond)

You will need to do the following:

1. Heat your oven to 350
2. Melt your cream cheese and cheese
3. Mix in the flour and your egg.
4. Get a baking sheet and line it with parchment paper.
5. Flatten your mixture on top of the sheet.
6. Sprinkle your garlic on the mixture.
7. Bake for twenty minutes.

Nutritional information:

Serving size is one.

- Calories-56
- Protein-3.6 grams
- Fat-4.5 grams
- Fiber-0.2 grams
- Carbs-0.8 grams

Strawberries to the rescue!

You will need 5 minutes for this

You will get one serving from this

You will need:

- 2/3 of a cup of water
- Half a cup of strawberries (you can use either use frozen or fresh)
- Half a teaspoon of vanilla extract
- A third of a cup of coconut milk that is unsweetened.

What you need to do:

1. Place all of the ingredients in your blender.
2. Blend it all until smooth.
3. Pour in a glass.

Nutritional information:

- Calories-149
- Carbs-8 grams
- Protein-6 grams
- Fiber-2 grams
- Fat-11 grams

Chia smoothie

You will need 5 minutes for this

You will get 4 serving from this

You will need:

- A single cup of blueberries (frozen)
- A half-cup of coconut cream
- A single cup of yogurt (use Greek and full fat)
- 2 tablespoons of coconut oil
- A single cup of almond milk that is unsweetened
- 2 tablespoons of sweetener (we're going with Swerve)
- 2 tablespoons of chia seeds (ground)

What you need to do:

1. Using a blender add all of your ingredients before blending until it is smooth.
2. Pour into glasses.

Nutritional information:

- Calories-249
- Fat-21.07 grams
- Fiber-3.55 grams
- Carbs-7.71 grams
- Protein-6.23 grams

Protein smoothie

You will need 5 minutes for this

You will get one serving from this

You will need:

- A single cup of ice
- Half of an avocado
- A single cup of spinach that's fresh
- 10 drops or 12 drops of Stevia Peppermint Sweet Drops (sweet leaf liquid drops)
- A single scoop of whey protein powder
- A half-cup of almond milk that is unsweetened
- A quarter teaspoon of peppermint extract

What you need to do:

1. Place everything but the drops, extract, and ice in the blender and blend.
2. Add the extract, ice, and drops.
3. Blend until its thick.

Nutritional information:

- Calories-293
- Fat-15 grams
- Carbs-11 grams
- Fiber- 7 grams
- Protein-28 grams

Blueberry smoothie

You will need 11 minutes for this

You will get one serving from this

You will need:

- A single cup of coconut milk
- A single teaspoon of vanilla extract
- A single teaspoon of coconut oil
- A quarter cup of blueberries

What you need to do:

1. Using a blender, blend until everything is smooth.

Nutritional information:

- Calories-215
- Fat-10 grams
- Carbs-7 grams
- Protein-23 grams
- Fiber-3 grams

Spinach smoothie

You will need 5 minutes for this

You will get one serving from this

You will need:

- 4 ice cubes
- A single tablespoon of mint (fresh)
- Half of a cup of cucumber (you will need to peel it before seeding it)
- A single cup of water (make sure it is filtered)
- A single cup of spinach (fresh)
- 4 ounces of coconut milk (canned and full fat)
- A single scoop of whey protein (grass-fed and naturally nourished)

What you need to do:

1. Get a blender.
2. Blend.
3. When smooth, pour in a glass.

Nutritional information:

- Calories-360
- Fat-24 grams
- Protein-27 grams
- Carbs-10 grams

Almond smoothie

You will need 5 minutes for this

You will get one serving from this

You will need:

- A single tablespoon of almond butter
- A single pinch of cinnamon
- A single teaspoon of vanilla extract
- A few ice cubes
- A single cup of almond milk (unsweetened)
- A single scoop of whey protein (use grass-fed and make sure that it is naturally nourished)

What you need to do:

1. Combine everything in a blender but the whey protein.
2. Once it's nice and mixed whip in your protein only for a moment to incorporate.

Nutritional information:

- Calories-255
- Fat-14 grams
- Carbs-7 grams

Protein- 29 grams

Avocado smoothie

You will need 2 minutes for this

You will get 2 servings from this

What you need:

- A single avocado (make sure it is ripe. You will peel and remove the pit)
- A cup and a third of water
- 2 tablespoons of sugar substitute (make sure its low carb)
- 2 to 3 tablespoons of juice from a lemon
- Half of a cup of raspberries (unsweetened and frozen)

What you need to do:

1. Place all of your ingredients in a blender.
2. Blend your ingredients until they are smooth.
3. Pour into a glass.

Nutritional value:

- Calories-227
- Fat-20 grams
- Fiber-8.8 grams
- Carbs-12.8 grams

Protein-2.5 grams

Pumpkin smoothie

You will need 5 minutes for this

You will get one serving with this

You will need:

- 3 tablespoons of puree (use pumpkin)
- A single teaspoon of tea (use loose chai)
- A single teaspoon of vanilla (alcohol-free)
- 3/4 of a cup of coconut milk (full fat)
- Half of a cup of avocado (use frozen)
- Half a teaspoon of pumpkin pie spice
- Half of an avocado (fresh. If fresh isn't available you can use frozen)

What you need to do:

1. Get a blender.
2. Add everything but avocado to the blender.
3. Blend until everything is smooth.
4. Add your avocado and blend.
5. Keep blending until broken apart.
6. Serve with the spice on top.

Nutritional information:

- Calories-726
- Fat-69.8 gram
- Fiber-8.2 grams
- Carbs-19.5 grams
- Protein-5.5 grams

Tumeric time!

You will need 5 minutes for this

You will get one serving for this

You will need:

- A single tablespoon of turmeric (use ground)
- 6.7 ounces of coconut milk (use full fat)
- A single teaspoon of cinnamon (use ground)
- 6.7 ounces of almond milk (unsweetened)
- A single teaspoon of granulated sweetener.
- A single tablespoon of chia seeds for the top of the smoothie
- A single tablespoon of coconut oil
- A single teaspoon of ginger (ground)

What you need to do:

1. Get a blender.
2. Place all of the ingredients in the blender, except chia seeds.
3. Add some ice if needed.
4. Blend until everything is smooth.
5. Sprinkle chia seeds to the top.

Nutritional information:

- Calories- 600
- Fat-56 grams
- Carbs-6 grams
- Protein-7 grams

Sausage sandwich

You will need 10 minutes for this

You will get one serving from this

What you need:

- A single tablespoon of cream cheese
- 2 sausage patties
- A single egg
- 2 tablespoons of cheddar (sharp)
- A quarter of a medium avocado (sliced)
- A quarter of a teaspoon to a half of a teaspoon of sriracha.

What you need to do:

1. Get a skillet.
2. Turn your heat to medium.
3. Cook sausages as the packet says to.
4. Set aside.
5. Mix your cheese with your sriracha.
6. Set it to the side.
7. Cook your egg into a small omelet.
8. Fill the omelet with cheese mix and assemble your sandwich

Nutritional information:

- Calories- 603
- Fat- 54 grams
- Protein-22 grams
- Carbs-7 grams

A taste of Italy omelet style

You will need 10 minutes for this

You will get 2 servings from this

What you need:

- Half a dozen eggs (six)
- 2 tablespoons of olive oil
- A single tablespoon of basil (fresh and chopped)
- 5 ounces of mozzarella cheese (fresh and diced)
- 3 tomatoes (cherry. Cut them in half)

What you need to do:

1. Get a bowl.
2. Crack your eggs into the bowl.
3. Add salt and pepper for taste.
4. Whisk with a fork and do it well. This lets the ingredients combine.
5. Add in your basil.
6. Stir.
7. Get a large frying pan.
8. Heat oil in the pan.
9. Fry your tomatoes for a few minutes.
10. Pour the egg mixture on the tomatoes.
11. After the batter has become slightly firm, add your cheese.
12. Turn down your heat and let your omelet set.
13. It is now ready to eat.

Nutritional information:

- Calories-534
- Fat-43 grams
- Fiber-1 gram
- Carbs-4 grams
- Protein-33 grams

Pancakes

You will need 12 minutes for this

You will get 4 servings from this

What you need:

- 2 ounces of cream cheese
- 2 eggs
- A single teaspoon of granulated sugar substitute
- Half of a teaspoon of cinnamon

What you need to do:

1. Put all of your ingredients in a blender.
2. Blend until its smooth.
3. Let it sit for 2 minutes.
4. Pour a quarter of the mix into a pan that is hot. The pan needs to be greased with butter.
5. Cook for 2 minutes .
6. It should be golden.
7. Flip it.
8. Cook another minute.
9. Repeat until the mix is gone.

Nutritional information:

- Calories-344
- Fat-29 grams
- Carbs-3 carbs
- Protein-17 carbs

Muffins

You will need only one minute for this

You will get one serving for this

You will need:

- A single egg
- A pinch of baking soda
- A pinch of salt
- 2 tablespoons of flour (coconut)

What you need to do:

1. Get a large coffee mug.
2. Grease it with oil (coconut) or butter if you don't have oil.
3. Mix everything together.
4. Make sure you have no lumps.
5. Cook in the microwave on high.
6. Do this for 45 seconds to a single minute.
7. Cut in two pieces, and you have a muffin.

Nutritional information:

- Calories-113
- Fat-6 grams
- Fiber-3 grams
- Protein-7 grams
- Carbs- 5 grams

Hearty breakfast

You will need 15 minutes for this

You will get one serving for this

You will need:

- 2 eggs (organic, pastured, large)
- 4 bacon strips (pastured, and uncured)
- A single avocado (large. You need to peel it before cutting it in slices)
- A quarter teaspoon of sea salt

What you need to do:

1. Put the bacon and avocado in a non-toxic ceramic frying pan on medium heat.
2. Cook three minutes before flipping both.
3. Remove both from the pan and place to the side.
4. Make sure that they are keeping warm.
5. Leave the drippings in the pan.
6. Crack your eggs into the pan.
7. You will be frying them for two to three minutes.
8. Flip your egg and fry until it is how you like.

Nutritional information:

- Calories-313
- Fat-26 grams
- Fiber- 6 grams
- Carbs-2.6 grams
- Protein-13 grams

Avocado lemon smoothie

You will need minutes for this

You will get servings from this

What you need:

- A simple cup of water that is cold
- Half of a cup of cilantro
- A single cup of spinach (use baby spinach)
- A single cup of avocado (use frozen)
- Peeled ginger (use a one-inch ginger)
- Half of a peeled lemon to one whole peeled lemon
- 3/4 of an English cucumber (it needs to be peeled)

What you need to do:

1. Get a blender that is high speed.
2. Add everything in the blender.
3. Blend until everything is smooth.
4. You need to store it in an airtight container.
5. It will last no longer than three days.

Nutritional information:

- Calories-148
- Fat-11 grams
- Fiber-6 grams
- Carbs- 13 grams
- Protein-2 grams

Cucumber smoothie

You will need 5 minutes for this

You will get 2 servings from this

What you need:

- 8 ounces of water
- A single cup of sliced cucumber
- 2 ounces of avocado (make sure it is ripe)
- A half teaspoon of liquid stevia (lemon)
- A single teaspoon of lemon juice
- 2 teaspoons of Green Tea powder (use match)
- Half a cup of ice
- A single teaspoon of juice from a lemon

What you need to do:

1. Pour your powder and water into a blender.
2. Blend to let the two combine.
3. Add the rest of your ingredients and blend. You should blend on high until it has become smooth.

Nutritional information:

- Calories-69
- Fat-4.6 grams
- Fiber- 3.4 grams
- Protein-2 grams
- Carbs-6.8 grams

Dragon fruit smoothie

You will need 5 minutes for this

You will get one serving from this

You will need:

- Half of a dragon fruit (small)
- Half of a cup of coconut milk
- A single galia melon wedge (small wedge)
- A single tablespoon of chia seeds
- 3 drops to 6 drops liquid stevia extract
- A single scoop of whey protein powder (vanilla)
- Try to find organic if you can for these ingredients

What you need to do:

1. Measure your ingredients and place them in a blender.
2. Pulse in your blender until smooth and ready to drink.

Nutritional information:

- Calories-403
- Fat-28.6 grams
- Protein-24.6
- Carbs-17 grams
- Fiber-4.9 grams

Egg smoothie

You will need 5 minutes for this

You will get one serving from this

You will need:

- A quarter cup of whipping cream (heavy)
- A half teaspoon of cinnamon
- A single egg (large one)
- 4 Cloves (ground)
- A single teaspoon of Erythritol

What you need to do:

1. Put all of your ingredients into a blender.
2. Blend.
3. If you do this for 60 seconds, you will get a bit of froth at the top.

Nutritional information:

- Calories-320
- Fat-30 grams
- Carbs-8 grams
- Fiber- 2 grams
- Protein-6 grams

Burrito

You will need 7minutes for this

You will get 1 serving from this (one burrito)

What you need:

- 2 eggs (use medium)
- A single tablespoon of butter
- 2 tablespoons of full fat cream

What you need to do:

1. Get a bowl.
2. Whisk the eggs in the bowl along with the cream.
3. Get a frying pan.
4. Melt your butter in the pan.
5. Pour in egg mix.
6. Swirl your frying pan until your burrito mixture is both thin and spread evenly.
7. Place a lid over the burrito pan.
8. Cook two minutes.
9. Lift burrito from pan.
10. Put on a plate.
11. If you choose to fill with veggies!

Nutritional information:

- Calories-331
- Fat-30 grams
- Carbs-1 gram
- Protein-11 grams

Let's get back to basics

You will need 10 minutes for this

You will get 2 servings from this

What you need:

- Half a dozen eggs (six)
- 3 ounces of butter
- 7 ounces of cheddar cheese (use shredded)

What you need to do:

1. Whisk your eggs. When they are frothy (slightly) and smooth, you can continue.
2. Blend in 3.5 ounces of cheddar (half)
3. Get a frying pan.
4. Melt your butter.
5. The pan needs to be hot for you to do this.
6. Pour in your egg mix.
7. Let it sit for a few moments.
8. Lower your heat.
9. Continue to cook until the egg mix has almost cooked through.
10. Add the rest of the cheese.
11. Fold omelet.
12. Place on a plate after removing from the stove.

Nutritional information:

- Calories-897
- Fat-80 grams
- Carbs-4 grams
- Protein-40 grams

Mocha smoothie

You will need 5minutes for this

You will get 3 servings from this

What you need:

- A single teaspoon of vanilla extract
- Half of a cup of coconut milk.
- A cup and a half of almond milk that is unsweetened
- 2 teaspoons of regular instant coffee crystals
- 3 tablespoons of a granulated stevia/erythritol blend
- 3 tablespoons of cocoa powder that is unsweetened
- A single avocado cut in half (the pit needs to be removed)

What you need to do:

1. Place everything in a blender except the avocado.
2. Blend it until it becomes smooth.
3. Add in your avocado by scooping it in.
4. Blend until smooth again.
5. Pour into 3 glasses.

Nutritional information:

- Calories-176
- Fat-16
- Carbs-10
- Fiber-6 grams
- Protein-3 grams

Chapter 4: Lunch Recipes

Lemon soup

You will need 15 minutes for this

You will get roughly 6 servings from this (possibly less)

What you need:

- 4 cups of water
- 2 tablespoons of lemon juice
- 2 cups of almond milk (unsweetened)
- ¾ of a cup of parmesan cheese
- 2.5 to 3 pounds of broccoli florets

What you need to do:

1. Get a large saucepan and then place your water and broccoli inside.
2. Cover the pan and cook on medium-high heat.
3. Do this until your broccoli is tender.
4. Reserve on the cups of the cooking liquid, but you can throw the rest away.
5. Add in half of the broccoli to a blender.
6. Add in the liquid you saved and the milk as well.
7. Blend until it's nice and smooth.
8. Return the mix to your pot and then add the parmesan along with your juice.
9. Heat it until it is hot.

Nutritional information:

- Calories-85
- Fat-3.1 grams
- Carbs-10.3 grams
- Protein-6.8 grams
- Fiber-4.0 grams

Caper salad

You will need 5 minutes for this

You will get 4 servings from this

You will need:

- Four ounces tuna (make sure that it is in olive oil)
- A single tablespoon of capers
- 2 tablespoons of creme fraiche
- Half a cup of mayo
- Half of a finely chopped leek
- Half a teaspoon of chili flakes

What you need to do:

1. Drain tuna.
2. Mix everything together.
3. Season

Nutritional information:

- Calories-271
- Fat-26 grams
- Carbs- 1 grams
- Protein 8 grams

Salmon with cucumber

You will need 20 minutes for this

You will get 4 servings from this

What you need for the Salmon:

- A single pound and a half of salmon (and it needs to be in pieces)
- 2 tablespoons of oil (use olive)
- 2 tablespoons of seasoning (use tendori)

What you need for the sauce:

- 3/4 of a cup of mayo
- 2 cloves of minced garlic
- Juice from half a lime
- Half of a cucumber (make sure that it is shredded)

What you need for your salad:

- 5 ounces of lettuce (use romaine)
- 3 scallions
- The juice from a lime
- A single bell pepper (use yellow)
- 2 avocados

What you need to do:

1. Heat your oven to 350.
2. Mix the seasoning with oil.
3. Cover your salmon with the mixture.
4. Bake for fifteen minutes minimum and twenty minutes maximum.
5. Your salmon should flake easily with a fork.
6. Mix everything together but the scallions, peppers, avocados, and lime juice. With the shredded cucumber, the water needs to be squeezed out.
7. Chop the remaining ingredients.
8. Place on your plate.
9. Over the top, drizzle your juice from the lime.
10. Next to them, place your salad and put the salmon on top.
11. Then top it with it the sauce.

Nutritional information:

- Calories-886
- Fat-76 grams
- Protein-38 grams
- Carbs-8 grams
- Fiber-9 grams

Pumpkin soup

You will need 20 minutes for this

You will get 6 servings for this

You will need:

- 15 ounces of puree (pumpkin)
- Half a teaspoon of pepper
- Half a teaspoon of salt
- 4 cups of broth (go with chicken)
- A single teaspoon of thyme (make sure it's fresh)
- Half a teaspoon of garlic powder
- Half a cup of heavy cream

What you need to do:

1. In a saucepan, combine everything but the heavy cream.
2. Stir, so they combine properly.
3. Bring to a boil.
4. Reduce heat and let it simmer for ten minutes.
5. Remove from heat before adding the cream.

Nutritional information:

- Calories-120
- Fat-9 grams
- Fiber-2 grams
- Carbs-7 grams
- Protein-2 grams

Let's grill some shrimp

You will need 40 minutes for this

You will get 4 servings for this

You will need:

- A single garlic clove that is small
- A single tablespoon of toasted pine nuts
- 2 tablespoons of oil (we're going with olive)
- A single tablespoon of lemon juice from a lemon
- Half of a cup of packed basil
- A single pound of peeled and deveined shrimp
- 2 tablespoons grated parmesan

What you need to do:

1. Get a blender.
2. Pulse all of your ingredients except the shrimp in blender.
3. Let the shrimp marinate in the mix.
4. Do this for 20 minutes. If you have time, do it overnight in your refrigerator.
5. Skewer your shrimp and grill.
6. You will do this over a medium-high heat until cooked thoroughly.
7. This should take 3 minutes for each side.

Nutritional information:

- Calories-184
- Fat-11 grams
- Carbs-2 grams
- Protein-18 grams

Egg roll with a twist

You will need 30 minutes for this

You will get 4 servings from this

You will need:

- A single pound of ground pork
- A single white diced onion
- A single teaspoon of ginger (grated)
- 2 minced garlic cloves
- 12 ounces of a coleslaw mix
- 2 teaspoons of apple cider vinegar
- 2 tablespoons of chopped green onion
- 2 tablespoons of sesame oil
- 3 tablespoons coconut aminos

What you need to do:

1. Get a large skillet.
2. Turn heat to medium.
3. Bown your pork
4. When it is cooked, you can set it to the side.
5. Be sure to discard all of the fat.
6. With the skillet, you just used heat your oil on medium heat.
7. Using the same skillet, heat the oil on medium heat.
8. Put the garlic, ginger, and onion in the skillet.

9. Do this until the onion is translucent and is fragrant.
10. Pour your coleslaw mix in along with the aminos and vinegar.
11. Stir well so it can combine.
12. Saute for five minutes. The cabbage should have reduced in size. Your carrots should also be softened.
13. Reincorporate your pork and stir so it can combine.
14. Saute for another minute.
15. Remove from heat.
16. Top with your onions.

Nutritional information:

- Calories-351
- Fat-15.8 grams
- Carbs-15.8 grams
- Fiber-2.6 grams
- Protein-38.2 grams

Baked fish with sauce

You will need 20 minutes for this

You will get 2 servings from this

What you need:

- A teaspoon of garlic paste
- Whitefish fillets (use 150 gram fish. You need 2 of them)
- A single tablespoon of oil (use olive)
- A single broccolini bunch
- A single lemon
- 100 grams of butter

What you need to do:

1. Preheat your oven to 428F.
2. Get a baking dish.
3. Line it with baking paper.
4. Finely grate the rind of the lemon.
5. Cut half of the lemon. They need to be in small segments.
6. Pat your fish dry.
7. Drizzle the fish with half of the rind and olive oil.
8. Bake for a minimum of twelve minutes and a maximum of fourteen. It should be cooked through. It should also be able to just fall apart.
9. Steam broccolini until its just tender. This should be done in a microwave for four minutes.

10. Drain it.
11. Place it to the side so it can dry.
12. Get a frying pan.
13. Turn the heat to medium.
14. Heat your butter for four minutes. It should be golden or almost golden.
15. Add the rest of the rind and your garlic.
16. Cook for another sixty seconds.
17. Stir in your segments of lemon and the broccolini.
18. Top the fish with your sauce and broccolini.

Nutritional information:

- Calories-476
- Fat-47 grams
- Fiber-2 grams
- Carbs-12 grams
- Protein- 19 grams

Subs

You will need 10 minutes for this

You will get 8 servings from this

What you need:

- 4 green onions (be sure to slice in half)
- 2 avocados (remove the pit, peel it and slice it)
- 2 leaves of lettuce (use iceberg)
- 9 ounces of ham (use Italian style)
- 5 and a half ounces of genoa salami
- 5 and a half of salami (use soppressata)
- 4 and a half ounces of prosciutto

What you need to do:

1. Place a slice a ham slice on a cutting board
2. Add a piece of prosciutto.
3. Add four pieces of salami.
4. Make a square shape with your layers.
5. Add some avocado (just a couple of slices)
6. Add a green onion piece.
7. Add a piece of lettuce to the far side of your meat stack that you have made.
8. Roll the ingredients into a roll.

Nutritional information:

- Calories-270
- Fiber-22 grams
- Fat-3.8 grams
- Carbs-6.3 grams
- Protein-18.6 grams

Tuna salad

You will need 10 minutes for this

You will get one serving from this

You will need:

- One sliced green onion
- 2 cups of greens (mixed)
- Half of a diced avocado
- A single diced tomato (use a large one)
- A quarter cup of chopped fresh mint
- A quarter cup fresh chopped parsley
- 10 large pitted kalamata olives
- A single can of chunk light tuna (make sure it is in water and drain it)
- A single small sliced zucchini (slice it lengthwise)
- A single tablespoon of balsamic vinegar
- A single tablespoon of extra virgin olive oil

What you need to do:

1. Get a skillet (cast iron).
2. Grill your zucchini slices. Do it on both sides in a sizzling hot skillet.
3. Remove from your pan.
4. Let it cool for a few moments.
5. Cut into pieces.
6. Get a bowl.
7. Put all of the ingredients in a bowl.
8. Stir it together.

Nutritional information:

- Calories-563
- Fat-30.9 grams
- Carbs-37.5 grams
- Protein- 41.8 grams
- Fiber-15 grams

Taco time

You will need 45 minutes for this

You will get 8 servings from this

You will need:

- A single pound of ground beef
- Half a dozen eggs (six and use large ones)
- A single cup of heavy cream
- 2 minced garlic cloves
- 3 tablespoons of taco seasoning
- A single cup cheese (shredded and cheddar)

What you need to do:

1. Preheat your oven to 350.
2. Get a pie pan that is 9 inches.
3. Grease the pan.
4. Get a skillet that is large.
5. Turn your heat to medium.
6. Brown ground beef until there is no pink left.
7. This should take approximately seven minutes. Make sure there are no clumps.
8. Add the seasoning and stir until it has been combined.
9. Reduce your heat to medium-low. Cook for another few minutes longer.
10. Your sauce should be thickened.

11. Place your beef in the pan before spreading it out.
12. Get a bowl.
13. Combine the garlic, cream, and eggs.
14. If you like salt and pepper, add a sprinkle.
15. Pour the mix over your beef.
16. Sprinkle the cheese over the top.
17. Bake for a half-hour.
18. The center needs to be set, and your cheese should be browned.
19. Remove from oven.
20. Let your dish sit for five minutes.
21. Slice and you are ready to eat.

Nutritional information:

- Calories-370
- Fat-27.8 grams
- Carbs-2.14 grams
- Protein-24.1 grams

Cabbage plate

You will need 10 minutes for this

You will get 2 servings for this

What you need:

- 10 ounces of bacon
- 2 ounces of butter
- A single pound of green cabbage

You will need to do the following:

- Chop your ingredients into small pieces (not butter)
- Get a skillet.
- Fry your bacon over medium heat until it is crisp.
- Add the cabbage and butter .
- Fry it until it has become golden and soft.

Nutritional information:

- Calories-850
- Carbs-9 grams
- Fiber-6 grams
- Fat- 79 grams
- Protein-21 grams

Let's get those veggies!

You will need a half an hour for this

You will get 2 servings from this

What you need:

- A third of an eggplant
- Half a lemon(you want the juice)
- 10 olives (black)
- Half of a zucchini
- 5 ounces of cheese (use cheddar) a quarter of a cup of olive oil
- Half a cup of mayo
- A single ounce of a leafy green
- 2 tablespoons of almonds

What you need to do:

1. Slice your eggplant into slices a half-inch thick.
2. Do the same with your zucchini. The slices should also be lengthwise.
3. Sprinkle salt on both sides of the vegetables you have cut and then let them sit for a maximum of ten minutes and a minimum of 5.
4. Preheat your oven to 450 degrees.
5. Use paper towels to pat your vegetables until dry on the surface.
6. Get a baking sheet.
7. Line it with parchment paper.

8. Brush olive oil over the top before sprinkling pepper over them to add flavor.
9. Bake for fifteen minutes minimum and twenty at the maximum.
10. They should appear golden Bryan on both sides. Remember to flip halfway through.
11. Place on a plate and pour the juice and oil over the top.
12. Serve with the rest of your vegetables and arrange them how you like them.

Nutritional information:

- Calories-1013
- Fat-99 grams
- Fiber-6 grams
- Carbs-9 grams
- Protein-21 grams

Chicken plate

You will need 5 minutes for this

You will get two servings from this

You will need:

- A single pound of rotisserie chicken
- 2 ounces of lettuce
- 7 ounces of cheese (use feta)
- 2 tomatoes
- 10 olives (black)
- A third of a cup of olive oil

What you need to do:

1. Slice your veggies and put them on a plate
2. Add the other ingredients together on the plate.
3. Place the oil in a small dish in the middle, or pour over the top.
4. You can sprinkle pepper and salt over the top if you like.

Nutritional information:

- Calories-1194
- Fiber-2 grams
- Fat-102 grams
- Carbs-3 grams
- Protein-62 grams

Mushroom plate

You will need 15 minutes for this

You will get 2 servings from this

You will need:

- 10 olives (use green)
- 10 ounces of cheese (you need to use halloumi)
- 10 ounces of mushrooms
- 3 ounces of butter

What you need to do:

1. Your mushrooms need to be clean.
2. Rinse them and make sure that they are before trimming them.
3. Cut them into pieces.
4. Heat up a dollop of butter in a pan for frying.
5. Turn the heat to medium.
6. Fry your mushrooms for no longer than five minutes and no less than three minutes. They should be a golden brown color.
7. While your frying your mushrooms, fry your cheese on the other side of the pan.
8. You can fry the cheese on both sides for a couple of minutes.
9. Stir the mushrooms occasionally while they are frying.
10. The heat should be lowered toward the end.

11. When your ready to eat, place the olives around
    the cheese.

Nutritional information:

- Calories-830
- Fat-74 grams
- Fiber-2 grams
- Carbs-7 grams
- Protein-36 grams

Italian time

You will need 5 minutes for this

You will get two servings from this

You will need:

- 7 ounces of mozzarella cheese (make sure it's fresh)
- 10 olives (green)
- A third of a cup of olive oil
- 2 tomatoes
- 7 ounces of sliced prosciutto

What you need to do:

1. Arrange all of the items on your plate in any fashion you like.
2. Place the oil in a small dish and place it in the center.

Nutritional information:

- Calories-822
- Fiber-3 grams
- Carbs-4 grams
- Protein-40 grams
- Fat-69 grams

Eggplant plate

You will need 10 minutes for this

You will get 2 servings from this

What you need:

- A single eggplant
- 10 ounces cheese (use halloumi)
- 3 ounces of butter
- 10 olives (black)

What you need to do:

1. Cut your eggplant in half (lengthwise).
2. Cut into slices. (Go for a half-inch in thickness).
3. Heat butter in a pan for frying.
4. Place eggplant alone on one side and the cheese on the other.
5. On a medium-high heat fry for seven minutes maximum and five minimum.
6. Remember to flip the cheese after three minutes. It should be golden brown on both sides.
7. Stir the vegetables once every few minutes.
8. When you are ready to eat, place your olives around the dish.

Nutritional information:

- Calories-829
- Fiber-8 grams
- Fat-72 grams
- Carbs-11 grams
- Protein-32 grams

Avocado, anyone?

You will need 10 minutes for this

You will get one serving for this

You will need:

- A single avocado (organic)
- A single ounce of goat cheese (use soft and fresh)
- 2 ounces of smoked salmon (wild-caught)
- 2 tablespoons of olive oil (use organic and make sure that it is extra virgin)
- The juice from a single lemon
- a pinch of salt (use celtic sea salt)

What you need to do:

1. Cut your avocado in two pieces and remove the pit.
2. In a food processor, add the rest of your ingredients until they have been chopped coarsely.
3. Place mixture inside your avocado.

Nutritional information:

- Calories-525
- Fat-48 grams
- Carbs-4 grams
- Protein-19 grams

Egg soup

You will need minutes for this

You will get one serving from this

What you need:

- A single cup and a half of chicken broth
- A half cube of chicken bouillon
- A single tablespoon of bacon fat
- 2 eggs (use large ones)
- A single teaspoon of chili garlic paste

What you need to do:

1. Get a pan and place it on your stove before setting your heat to medium-high.
2. Add the broth, fat, and bouillon cube.
3. Bring your broth to boiling and stir.
4. Add your paste and stir.
5. Turn off your stove.
6. Get a bowl.
7. Beat your eggs in the bowl before you pour it in the broth.
8. Stir well.
9. Let sit for a moment so that it will cook.

Nutritional information:

- Calories-289
- Fat-23.24 grams
- Carbs-2.92 grams
- Protein-15.3 grams

Queso soup

You will need 35 minutes for this

You will get 4 servings from this

What you need:

- A single tablespoon of taco seasoning
- A single pound of chicken breast
- A single tablespoon of avocado oil 3 cups of broth (use chicken)
- 2 cans Rotel that are ten ounces with green chiles (diced)
- 8 ounces of cream cheese
- Half of a cup of heavy cream

What you need to do:

1. Get a pot or a dutch oven that is cast iron.
2. Turn your heat to medium.
3. Heat the oil.
4. Stir your Rotel into the pot.
5. Stir the seasoning in the pot.
6. Cook for a single minute.
7. Add in the chicken.
8. Add in your broth.
9. Cover your pan.
10. You will need to simmer for 25 minutes.
11. Remove your chicken and then proceed to shred it.

12. Set the chicken to the side.
13. Stir in your heavy cream.
14. Stir in your cream cheese.
15. When the cheese has melted, put the chicken back in the pot.
16. Season with salt and pepper if you so choose.

Nutritional information:

- Calories-491
- Fat-37.6 grams
- Protein-33.1 grams
- Carbs-9.6 grams

Smoked salmon

You will need 20 minutes for this

You will get 6 servings from this

What you need:

- 7 ounces of salmon (smoked)
- The zest from half of a lemon)
- 8 ounces of cream cheese
- 4 tablespoons of dill (fresh)
- 5 and an additional 1/3 tablespoons of mayo
- 2 ounces of lettuce

What you need to do:

1. Cut your salmon into pieces that are small.
2. Combine all of your ingredients in a bowl.
3. Let it sit for 15 minutes.
4. This lets the flavors develop.
5. Place on a lettuce leaf.

Nutritional information:

- Calories-330
- Fat-26 grams
- Protein- 23 grams
- Carbs-3 grams

Butter shrimp

You will need 25 minutes for this

You will get 4 servings for this

You will need:

- A single pound of raw shrimp (it will need to be large, wild-caught and you will need to devein it and peel it)
- 3 tablespoons of water
- Half a dozen sprigs of oregano (it will need to be fresh)
- A single cup of ghee (you should go for grass-fed)
- A single bay leaf
- A single zest from a lemon

What you need to do:

1. Get yourself a pan.
2. Bring water to a boil. To do so, your heat should be high.
3. Reduce your heat to medium before whisking in the ghee.
4. Whisk constantly.
5. Your sauce should become smooth, and the texture should be even.
6. Add the rest of your ingredients except water and sprinkle with salt.
7. Stir, so the shrimp gets coated.

8. Lay them evenly in your pan.
9. Bring the liquid in the pan up to a light simmer. Your heat should now be medium-low.
10. Cook your shrimp for five minutes. Make sure it's cooked all the way through and pink.
11. Serve with a little sauce and dill.

Nutritional information:

- Calories-304
- Fat-27 grams
- Carbs-5 grams
- Protein- 13 grams

Baked salmon

You will need 15 minutes for this

You will get 4 servings from this

What you need for the Salmon:

- 2 pounds of salmon
- 4 tablespoons of pesto (green)

What you need for the sauce:

- A single cup of mayo
- Half of a cup of yogurt (make sure that it is full fat and Greek)
- 4 tablespoons of pesto (green)

What you need to do:

1. Place your salmon in a baking dish that is greased.
2. Be sure its skin side down.
3. Spread the pesto over the top.
4. Bake for half an hour at 400 degrees.
5. The fish should flake easily with a fork.
6. Stir all of the sauce ingredients together.

Nutritional information:

- Calories-1037
- Fat-90 grams
- Fiber-0 grams
- Protein-50 grams
- Carbs-3 grams

Tomato soup

You will need 15 minutes for this

You will get six servings from it

What you need:

- A stick of unsalted butter
- 8 ounces of cream cheese
- 5 cups of tomato puree (you will get this by blending fresh tomato chunks (minus the stems))
- One handful of basil leaves (fresh)
- If you like add salt and pepper for tasting

What you need to do:

1. Puree the tomatoes to get five cups (an estimate to help you is that this would be about 4 large tomatoes and around a pint of cherry tomatoes)
2. Get a saucepan.
3. Pour the puree into the pan.
4. Add the cream cheese and butter.
5. Heat to a simmer and cook until both the butter and cream cheese melt.
6. Pour the soup back into your blender.
7. Add your basil.
8. Be sure that you are venting the lid as this is a hot liquid.
9. Puree till smooth.

Nutritional information:

- Calories-287
- Fat-28 grams
- Carbs-6 grams
- Protein-3 grams
- Fiber-1 gram

Salad on the go

You will need 10 minutes for this

You will get a single serving from this

What you need:

- A single avocado
- A single ounce of bell peppers. For this recipe, you should use red.
- A single ounce of cherry tomatoes
- A single carrot
- ½ of a scallion (make sure that it is sliced)
- A single ounce of leafy greens
- 4 ounces of rotisserie chicken or salmon that has been smoked (wherever your preference lies)
- ¼ of a cup of mayo or olive oil (wherever your preference lies)

What you need to do:

1. Chop the vegetables or shred them.
2. Get a jar.
3. Put the leafy greens at the bottom.
4. Add the other ingredients in layers.
5. Add the chicken or salmon to the top.
6. Add the mayo or oil.

This is fun to play around with. You could use eggs or tuna; this is perfect for women with a busy lifestyle.

Nutritional information:

- Calories-1133
- Fat-84 grams
- Fiber-17 grams
- Protein-75 grams
- Carbs-11 grams

Salmon plate

You will need 5 minutes for this

You will get 2 servings from this

What you need:

- 2 avocados
- Salt and pepper if you like for flavor and taste
- ½ of a cup of mayo
- 7 ounces of smoked salmon

What you will need to do:

- Split your avocados in half.
- Remove the pit before scooping the rest out with a spoon.
- Cut the leftover avocado (what you scooped out. The good stuff not the pit) into pieces.
- Place the pieces on a plate.
- Add your salmon to the plate and a dollop of mayo.
- Sprinkle the salt and pepper over the top.

Nutritional information:

Per serving.

- Calories-1037
- Protein-65 grams
- Fat-82 grams
- Fiber-13 grams
- Carbs- 2 grams

Slaw bowl

You will need 15 minutes for this

You will get 4 servings from this

What you need:

- A single teaspoon of avocado oil
- A single pound of ground beef
- 2 teaspoons of toasted sesame oil
- A quarter of a cup of green onions
- 1 teaspoon of sea salt
- A quarter of a cup of black pepper
- 4 cups of shredded coleslaw mix
- 3 tablespoons of ginger (fresh)
- 4 minced garlic cloves
- A quarter cup of coconut aminos
- A quarter cup of green onions

What you need to do:

1. In a large saute pan, you will need to heat your avocado oil on a heat that has been set to medium-high.
2. Add ginger and garlic.
3. Saute for a minute.
4. The smell should be fragrant for you.
5. Add the beef and season.
6. Cook between seven and ten minutes. The meat should be browned at this point.

7. Reduce the heat to medium.
8. Add the coconut and coleslaw mix and stir.
9. Cover it and cook for five minutes.
10. Remove from the heat and stir in your toppings
    (the sesame oil and onions)

Nutritional information:

One serving is 1 ½ cups (this would be the whole
meal). If you have it with something else (like a side
dish), it's one cup for a serving.

- Calories-457
- Fat-31 grams
- Protein-33 grams
- Carbs- 9 grams
- Fiber- 2 grams

Grilled steak

You will need 17 minutes for this

You will get around 6 servings to 8 servings with this

What you need for the sauce:

- A single clove of garlic
- A single tablespoon of oregano (fresh)
- ½ of a teaspoon of salt
- 4 tablespoons of oil (olive)
- ¼ of a teaspoon of pepper
- ¼ of a teaspoon of pepper flakes (red ones)
- A single tablespoon of lime juice (fresh)
- 3 diced avocados
- 3 tablespoons of vinegar (used red wine)

What you need for the meat:

- 2 pounds of flank steak
- Pepper for seasoning
- Salt for seasoning

What you need to do:

1. Heat a grill to medium-high heat or to 400 degrees.
2. Add all of the ingredients for the sauce to a food processor and blend until everything is smooth.
3. Get yourself a bowl.

4. Add the avocado and the sauce you blended.
5. Toss lightly, so it gets coated but not hard enough to crush the avocado.
6. Take a room temperature flank steak and season both sides with pepper and salt.
7. Place the steak on the grill and cook for a maximum of six minutes on each side and a minimum of four minutes.
8. Remove from your grill and let cool for a few minutes.
9. Slice the steak and drizzle the top with sauce or serve it on the side.

Nutritional information:

The serving size for this recipe is one steak (5 ounces) and sauce

- Calories-444
- Fat-32 grams
- Fiber-5 grams
- Protein-34 grams

Carbs-7 grams

Chapter 5: Dinner Recipes

Pork

You will need 35 minutes for this recipe

You will get 2 servings from this

What you need:

- A single pound of pork tenderloin
- A quarter cup of oil
- 3 medium shallots (chop them finely)

What you need to do:

1. Slice your pork into thick slices (go for about a half-inch thick).
2. Chop up your shallots before placing them on a plate.
3. Get a cast-iron skillet and warm up the oil
4. Press your pork into your shallots on both sides. Press firmly to make sure that they stick.
5. Place the slices of pork with shallots into the warm oil and then cook until it's done. The shallots may burn, but they will still be fine.
6. Make sure the pork is cooked through thoroughly.

Nutritional information:

- Calories-519
- Fat-36 grams
- Protein-46 grams
- Carbs-7 grams

Garlic shrimp

You will need 20 minutes for this

You will get 3 servings for this

What you need:

- 2 minced garlic cloves
- 2 whole garlic cloves
- The juice from half a lemon
- 2 tablespoons of oil (olive)
- 2 tablespoons of butter
- ¾ pounds of either small or medium shrimp (it needs to be both shelled and deveined)
- A quarter of a teaspoon of paprika
- A quarter of a teaspoon of pepper flakes (red ones)
- 2 tablespoons of parsley that is chopped.

What you have to do:

1. Sprinkle your shrimp with a teaspoon of salt (fine grain sea salt) and let it sit for ten minutes.
2. Get a skillet.
3. Heat the butter with olive oil over a heat that is medium-high.
4. Add the flakes and garlic.
5. Saute for half a minute.
6. Add your shrimp and cook until they have turned pink. This will take approximately two minutes. Stir constantly.

7. Add paprika and juice from the lemon.
8. Cook for another sixty seconds.

Nutritional information:
Per serving
- Calories-260
- Fat-18 grams
- Carbs-none
- Protein-24 protein

Pork Chop

You will need 40 minutes for this

You will get 6 servings for this

You will need:

- A dozen pork chop (boneless and thin cut)
- 2 cups of spinach (you should use baby spinach for this)
- 4 cloves of garlic
- A dozen slices provolone cheese

You will need to do the following things:

1. Preheat your oven to a temperature of 350.
2. Press the garlic cloves using a garlic press. The cloves should go through the press and into a small bowl.
3. Spread the garlic that you have made onto one side of the pork chops.
4. Flip half a dozen chops while making sure the garlic side is down.
5. You should do this on a baking sheet that is rimmed.
6. Divide your spinach between the half dozen chops.
7. Fold cheese slices in half.
8. Put them on top of the spinach.
9. Put a second pork chop on top of the first set, but this time make sure that the garlic side is up.

10. Bake for 20 minutes.

11. Cover each chop with another piece of cheese.

12. Bake another 15 minutes.

13. Your meat meter should be at 160 degrees when you check with a thermometer.

Nutritional information:

- Calories-436
- Fat-25 grams
- Carbs-2 grams
- Protein-47 grams

Citrus egg salad

You will need 10 minutes for this

You get 3 servings from this

What you need:

- Half a dozen eggs (6)
- A single teaspoon of mustard (go with Dijon)
- 2 tablespoons of mayo
- A single teaspoon of lemon juice

What you need to do:

1. Place the eggs gently in a medium saucepan.
2. Add cold water until your eggs are covered by an inch.
3. Bring to a boil.
4. You should do this for ten minutes. Remove from your heat and cool. Peel your eggs under running water that is cold .
5. Put your eggs in a food processor. Pulse until they are chopped.
6. Stir in condiments and juice.

Nutritional information:

- Calories-222
- Fat-19 grams
- Protein-13 grams
- Carbs-1 gram

Chowder

You will need 40 minutes

You will get 4 servings from this

You will need:

- A single tablespoon of butter
- 5 minced garlic cloves
- An entire head of cauliflower (cut it into florets that are small)
- Half of a teaspoon of oregano (use dried)
- Half a cup of carrots that have been diced
- Half a cup of onions that have been diced
- A cup and a half of broth (use vegetable)
- A quarter cup of cream cheese

What you need to do:

1. Get a soup pot.
2. Heat your butter.
3. Add garlic and onions.
4. Saute for a few moments.
5. Add the rest of the ingredients to the pot.
6. Bring to a boil.
7. Slow the heat and put it on a simmer.
8. Cook for 15 minutes.
9. Shut off the flame.
10. Use a hand blender to blend the soup partly in the pot.
11. Switch the flame back on.

12.   Add a cup of broth.

13.   Add the cream cheese.

14.   Simmer for 10 minutes and switch off the flame again.

Nutritional information:

Per serving

- Calories-143
- Fat-8.4 grams
- Carbs-15.2 grams
- Protein-4.5 grams

Avocado salad

You need 10 minutes for this

You get one serving from this

What you need:

* 3 ounces of cooked and shredded chicken breast
* A single stalk of celery
* A single tablespoon of diced red onions
* A third of a cup of sour cream
* A single avocado (go with a medium)

What you need to do:

1. Cook the chicken on low heat until it is fully cooked.
2. Shred it using forks.
3. Get a bowl.
4. Place your celery, chicken, and onion inside to combine.
5. Cut your avocado and put your avocado.
6. Scoop some of the avocado out before putting it in the bowl.
7. Add the sour cream.
8. Toss everything well.
9. Put the mix back in the avocado halves.

Nutritional information:

* Calories-570
* Protein-29 grams
* Fat-45 grams
* Carbs-5 grams

Tex plate

You will need 20 minutes for this

You will get 6 servings for this

You will need:

- ⅔ of a pound of ground beef
- 4 tablespoons of olive oil
- 2 tablespoons of water. It needs to be cold.
- A single tablespoon of seasoning (go with tex mex on this one)
- A single ounce of sliced pepper jack cheese (for a kick)
- 2 avocados
- 2 tablespoons of jalapenos (they need to be pickled)
- A third of a cup of mayo
- 2 ounces arugula lettuce

What you need to do:

1. Mix the water, meat, and seasoning.
2. Form one burger per serving.
3. Brush half of the olive oil that you have around each burger that you have.
4. Fry them for four minutes on each side. The burger should be light pink or cooked entirely through.
5. Place your burger on a plate with all the other vegetables and cheese.
6. Drizzle the oil over the top of everything.

Nutritional information:

- Calories-1067
- Fiber-15 grams
- Carbs- 7 grams
- Protein-39 grams
- Fat-95 grams

Eggs and tuna

You will need 10 minutes for this

You will get 2 servings of this

What you need:

- 2 tablespoons of olive oil
- 2 tablespoons of capers that are small
- 2 ounces of tomatoes (cherry)
- 2 ounces lettuce
- 4 ounces of tuna (it needs to be in olive oil and drained)
- Half of a lemon you want the zest and juice from it
- A third of a cup of celery stalks that have been chopped
- Half a cup of mayo
- Half of a red onion
- A single teaspoon of mustard (use dijon)

For your eggs:

- 4 ounces
- 2 teaspoons of vinegar (white wine vinegar)
- A single teaspoon of salt

What you need to do for this:

1. Mix your tuna with the other ingredients on the first list. Don't mix the lettuce or tomatoes, however.

2.   Bring water in a pot to a light boil.

3.   Add in the vinegar and salt before stirring the water. You should be making a swirl with your spoon.

4.   Crack the egg into the water while it's moving.

5.   Do this one at a time.

6.   Let it simmer for three minutes.

7.   Remove from your water using a spoon that is slotted.

8.   Use the lettuce and tomatoes when you're ready to eat and pour the olive oil over the top.

Nutritional information:

- Calories-765
- Fiber-3 grams
- Carbs-6 grams
- Fat- 69 grams
- Protein-29 grams

Fried chicken

You will need 15 minutes for this

You will get 2 servings

You will need:

- 10 ounces of chicken thighs that are boneless
- 9 ounces of broccoli
- 3 and a half ounces of butter

What you need to do:

1. Rinse the broccoli.
2. Trim the broccoli as well.
3. Cut the broccoli into small pieces. This will include the stem.
4. Heat up a good part of the butter in a pan for frying.
5. Season your chicken with pepper and salt if you like.
6. Fry it over a heat that is medium for 5 minutes per side. It should be cooked through.
7. Add another helping of the butter and put the broccoli in the same pan you have been using and fry the broccoli for two minutes.
8. Season more (if you need to. If you don't, then leave it as is.), and then when you plate it serve it with the rest of the butter that you haven't used.

Nutritional information:

- Calories-733
- Fiber- 3 grams
- Fat-66 grams
- Carbs-5 grams
- Protein-29 grams

Ground beef plate

You will need 15 minutes for this

You will get 2 servings from this

You will need:

*   10 ounces of ground beef
*   3 and a half ounces of butter
*   9 ounces of green beans that are fresh

What you will need to do:

*   Rinse your green beans.
*   Trim them.
*   Heat up part of your butter in a pan for frying.
*   Brown your ground beef on a heat that is high until it is almost done.
*   Lower your heat and on the opposite side of the pan (next to the meat), add another portion of butter.
*   Fry your green beans for five minutes.
*   Stir your ground beef.
*   Season beans with salt and pepper if you wish.
*   Plate everything and serve with the rest of the butter.

Nutritional information:

*   Calories-694
*   Fat-60 grams
*   Fiber-3 grams
*   Carbs-5 grams
*   Protein-32 grams

Mac n cheese

You will need 4 minutes for this

You will get one serving from this

What you need:

- A single ounce of shredded cheddar cheese
- A single tablespoon of heavy cream
- ¾ of a cup of florets of cauliflower that are frozen

What you need to do:

1. Get a microwavable dish that has a lid.
2. Microwave it covered for a minute.
3. Remove and chop the cauliflower. The pieces should be small.
4. Microwave for another 50 seconds and add the cheese.
5. Microwave 10 seconds.
6. Stir and stir in the heavy cream. This will form a sauce.

Nutritional information:

- Calories-191
- Fat-14.9
- Fiber-2
- Carbs-4.8
- Protein-9.4

Chicken with sauce

You will need 35 minutes for this

You will get 4 servings from this

You will need:

- 2 tablespoons of olive oil
- A single cup of keto dressing (use a keto honey mustard dressing)
- 4 chicken breasts that are skinless and boneless

You will need to do the following:

1. Combine the chicken and half of your dressing into a bowl.
2. Toss the chicken so it can get coated.
3. You will need to let it marinate in the fridge for an hour. If you have more time, you can do it up to 24 hours.
4. Preheat your oven to 350.
5. Heat the oil in a skillet that is oven-proof.
6. The heat should be medium-high.
7. When your pan is hot, you can add the chicken.
8. You will pan sear the chicken and brown it on both sides.
9. This will be 4 minutes on each side.
10. Pour the rest of the dressing on the chicken.
11. Transfer the skillet to the oven.
12. Bake 20 minutes.

13.   The chicken should be cooked all the way through, but if not, cook longer.

Nutritional information:

- Calories-242
- Fat-9.5 grams
- Protein-34 grams
- Carbs-1 gram

Chili pot

You will need an hour and five minutes for this

You will get 6 servings from this

What you will need:

- A single tablespoon and a half of avocado oil
- 2 pounds of pork shoulder (be sure to cut it into half a dozen pieces (6))
- A single cup and a half of salsa verde (herdez is a good brand)
- A single cup of broth (chicken broth)

What you need to do:

1. Rub your pork pieces with pepper and salt.
2. You will need an instant pot for this recipe.
3. Select the saute button.
4. Add the oil to the inner pot of the instant pot.
5. When the pot is hot, sear the pork pieces on all of the sides. Each side will take four minutes per side until they have browned.
6. In a bowl, combine your broth and salsa verde.
7. Stir.
8. Pour the mix over the pork.
9. Close and lock the lid of the instant pot.
10. Turn your pressure release handle to sealing.
11. Select pressure cooker manual on high pressure.
12. Set your timer for forty minutes.

13.   It will take a bit to start, but it will beep and then begin to countdown.
14.   Once your cooking time is done, you need to let the pressure naturally release for 10 minutes. This means let the pot sit for those minutes.
15.   Quick-release the remaining pressure. A good trick is to use a spoon made of wood to press the release handle to vent. You should keep your hands and face away from the steam, so you don't hurt yourself.
16.   When the pressure is released, remove your lid.
17.   Remove the pork and place on a plate.
18.   Shred the pork.
19.   Add the shredded pork back into the sauce that is still in the pot.
20.   Stir so that it can combine.

Nutritional information:

- Calories-342
- Fat-22 grams
- Fiber-2 grams
- Carbs-4 grams
- Protein-32 grams

Scallops

You will need 25 minutes for this

You will need 4 servings for this

You will need:

- 8 bacon slices that are cut in half (make sure that they are cut crosswise)
- 16 sea scallops
- Olive oil
- Toothpicks for the scallops

The steps you need to follow:

1. Preheat your oven to 425.
2. Pat your scallops with a paper towel, so they dry.
3. Remove any side muscles from the scallops.
4. Wrap a scallop in one of the bacon halves and stick a toothpick in it.
5. Repeat with the other 15 scallops.
6. Pour your olive oil over the scallops, and if you want to season them with salt and pepper. If you choose to do this, make sure that you are using kosher salt.
7. Arrange your scallops in a layer on a baking sheet that is prepared. Make sure that they are in a single layer.
8. You need to leave space between them, so make sure to do so.

9.   Bake fifteen minutes. The scallops should be tender and look opaque while your bacon should be cooked through.

10.   Make sure that they are hot when you serve them.

Nutritional information:

* Calories-224
* Fat-17 grams
* Carbs- 2 grams
* Protein-12 grams

Chicken casserole

You're going to need 25 minutes

You will get 8 servings out of this

You will need:

* 16 ounces of salsa
* 3 cups of shredded chicken
* 8 ounces of softened cream cheese
* 8 ounces of shredded cheese (use cheddar)
* ¾ of a teaspoon of chipotle pepper (ground)

What you need to do:

1. Preheat your oven to 400.
2. Grease a baking dish that is 9 by 13.
3. Get a bowl.
4. Combine all of the ingredients but only half of the cheese and half a teaspoon of pepper.
5. Mix it well.
6. Put the mix in the baking dish.
7. Top the dish with the leftover cheese and pepper.
8. Bake 20 minutes. It should be bubbly and hot.

Nutritional information:

* Calories- 319
* Fat-25 grams
* Fiber-1 gram
* Carbs-5 grams
* Protein-17 grams

Shrimp noodles

You will need 15 minutes for this

You will get 2 servings from this

You will need:

- A single tablespoon of olive oil
- The zest and juice from an entire lemon
- 2 zucchini that are medium in size
- 3 to 4 minced garlic cloves
- ¾ pounds of shrimp that are medium in size as well as peeled and deveined
- Fresh parsley that is chopped

What you will need to do:

1. With the zucchini, spiralize it on a setting of medium.
2. Set the spiralized veggie aside.
3. Get a skillet and put the heat to medium.
4. Add the lemon zest and juice along with olive oil to the pan.
5. Once the pan is warm, you can add the shrimp.
6. Cook the shrimp for a single minute on each side.
7. Add garlic and cook for a minute, making sure to stir.
8. Add the noodles (veggie noodles) and stir for 3 minutes. This is going to warm them up and cook them. If it helps use tongs.
9. Sprinkle with your parsley.
10. Serve right away.

Nutritional information:

- Calories-280

Tuna patties

You're going to need 15 minutes for this

You will get 6 servings for this

What you will need:

- One half of a cup of shredded cheese
- 2 eggs
- 4 ounces of pork rinds (we need them ground up into crumbs)
- 2 tablespoons of pico de gallo
- 2 cans of tuna that has been packed in water and 5 ounces each

What you will need to do:

1. Open your tuna and drain it.
2. Pulse your rinds in a food processor, so they become crumbs.
3. Get a bowl.
4. Mix all the ingredients until they have combined fully.
5. Separate the mixture so that you have six parts that you can make into patties.
6. Roll into six patties.
7. Fry in coconut oil for a few minutes on each of the sides.
8. When done, they should be golden brown.
9. Serve while they are warm.

Nutritional information:

One patty is one serving

- Calories-205
- Carbs-1.4 grams
- Fat- 11.5 grams
- Protein-22.6 grams

Meatballs

You will need 20 minutes for this

You will get 3 servings from this

You will need the following:

- A single teaspoon of garlic powder
- 3.5 ounces of mozzarella cheese
- 1.1 pounds of ground beef
- 3 tablespoons of parmesan cheese

What you will need to do:

1. Cut your cheese into cubes. Ideally, you want a single centimeter by a single centimeter.
2. Mix your dry ingredients with your ground beef.
3. Wrap the cubes that you made in the meat. You should get at least nine balls.
4. Pan-fry the meatballs.
5. Make sure to have a lid to capture the heat.
6. Make sure the cheese doesn't spill.

Nutritional information:

- Calories-444
- Fat-28 grams
- Protein-46 grams
- Carbs-2 grams

Chicken breasts

You will need a half-hour for this recipe

You're going to get 6 servings from this

What you need:

- A quarter of a cup of Greek yogurt
- Half of a cup of shredded mozzarella cheese
- 2 tablespoons of olive oil
- A pound and a half of chicken breasts. They need to be four-ounce portions
- A quarter cup of spinach. Frozen and drained, it should also be tightly packed.
- Half of a cup of thinly sliced artichoke hearts
- 4 ounces of softened cream cheese
- Half a teaspoon of divided salt
- A quarter of a teaspoon of divided pepper

What you need to do:

1. Pound your chicken breast to a single inch thick.
2. Use a sharp knife carefully and cut each breast down the middle. Do not cut all of the way. You are making a pocket.
3. Sprinkle the breasts with a quarter teaspoon of salt.
4. Sprinkle then with an eighth of a teaspoon of pepper.
5. Get a bowl.

6.   Combine everything except your oil and mix it thoroughly. You need the ingredients to combine thoroughly.

7.   Fill each breast with the mixture.

8.   Get a large skillet.

9.   Turn the heat to medium.

10.   In the skillet, add your oil and breasts.

11.   Cover the skillet and cook for 8 minutes on each side.

12.   Your chicken should reach 165 degrees when you check it with a meat thermometer.

13.   When it's the last few minutes of your cooking, add any leftover filling to the skillet, so it heats up.

14.   Server your chicken with cauliflower rice.

Nutritional information:

- Calories-288
- Fat-17 grams
- Protein-28 grams
- Carbs-2 grams

Cream cheese rollups

You will need 10 minutes for this

You will get 15 servings from this

You will need:

- 7 and a half teaspoons of chopped banana peppers
- 1.25 ounces of cream cheese
- 7 and a half teaspoons chopped red peppers
- 15 slices of salami

You will need to do the following:

1. Spread half a teaspoon of your cream cheese on each slice of your salami.
2. Spoon a single teaspoon of your red pepper on 5 slices of salami.
3. For the last five slices, you want to place half a teaspoon of each pepper onto the meat.
4. Fold each slice of meat over, so it looks like a taco.
5. If you need to keep it closed, use a toothpick.

Nutritional information:

One serving= one rollup

- Calories-50
- Fat-4.04 grams
- Fiber-0.06 grams
- Carbs-0.61 grams
- Protein-2.88 grams

Cheesy Quiche

You will need 35 minutes for this

You will get 9 servings from this

You will need:

- 7 eggs
- Half a cup of heavy cream
- 12 ounces of chopped broccoli
- 2 tablespoons of almond flour
- A cup and a third of cheese. (use sharp cheddar)
- Half of a cup of chopped red onions
- Half a teaspoon of ground mustard

What you need to do:

1. Preheat your oven to 350.
2. Spray a muffin tin (a small one) with a non-stick cooking spray.
3. Lightly flour the bottom.
4. Get a bowl.
5. Whisk your ingredients except the cheese, onions, and broccoli.
6. Stir in the broccoli cheese and onions.
7. Pour the mix into the baking tin.
8. Bake 40 minutes.
9. A knife should come out clean.

Nutritional information:

- Calories-183
- Fat-14.04 grams
- Fiber-0.58 grams
- Protein-9.06 grams
- Carbs-2.79 grams

Dinner box

You will need 15 minutes for this

You will get one serving from this

You will need:

- 2 tablespoons of almonds that are raw
- A single hard-boiled large egg
- A quarter cup of cherry tomatoes
- 2 ounces of turkey breast that are thinly sliced
- 4 pita bites crackers
- A single ounce of cubed and sharp cheddar cheese

What you need to do:

1. Get a meal prep container or a piece of tupperware that resembles one.
2. Place the ingredients in the container in any way you like.

Nutritional information:

- Calories-382
- Protein-23 grams
- Carbs-16 grams
- Fiber-3 grams
- Fat-25 grams

Elegant taco salad

You will need 20 minutes for this

You will get 6 servings from this

You will need:

- 8 ounces of chopped romaine lettuce
- A third of a cup of salsa
- A third of a cup of sour cream
- A single cubed medium avocado
- A single pound of ground beef
- A single teaspoon of avocado oil
- A cup and a third of halved grape tomatoes
- Half a cup of chopped green onions
- ¾ of a cup of shredded cheddar cheese
- 2 tablespoons of taco seasoning

You will need to do the following:

1. Get a skillet.
2. Heat your oil in the skillet at a heat that is high.
3. Add your beef.
4. Stir fry while making sure that you are breaking the pieces up.
5. You will need to stir fry for 10 minutes.
6. The beef should be browned, and the moisture should be evaporated.
7. Stir in the seasoning into the beef. Make sure it has combined well.
8. Get a bowl.

9.   Place all of the remaining ingredients in the bowl.
10.   Add the beef.
11.   Toss it all together.

Nutritional information:

Serving size is ⅙ of the recipe

- Calories-332
- Fat-25 grams
- Protein-20 grams
- Carbs-9 grams
- Fiber-4 grams

Loaded casserole

You will need an hour for this

You will get 8 servings from this

You will need:

- A single cup of cheddar cheese that is sharp
- A single head of cauliflower that is large and cut into florets
- A single cup of shredded cheese (use colby and monterey jack)
- 8 slices of bacon that has been fried crispy
- 6 tablespoons of chives that are fresh, chopped and divided
- Half of a cup of sour cream
- A single tablespoon of ranch seasoning
- Half a cup of mayo

You will need to do the following:

1. Preheat your oven to 370.
2. Get a baking dish that is 13 by 9 and spray with a non-stick cooking spray.
3. Get a large skillet.
4. Fry the bacon until it becomes crispy.
5. Crumble it and place to the side.
6. Steam the cauliflower for 20 minutes, as this will make it tender.
7. Get a bowl.

8.   Combine the seasoning, mayo, and sour cream before adding the cauliflower, 3 tablespoons of chives, half of your bacon, and a cup of the cheddar.

9.   Mix it all well.

10.   Pour the mixture into the baking dish.

11.   Top it with colby and monterey jack cheese.

12.   Top that with the other half of the bacon.

13.   Cover the dish with foil.

14.   Bake for 20 minutes.

15.   Take the foil off.

16.   Bake for another 10 minutes. Your cheese should be bubbly, and the color should be turning brown.

17.   Top with the other half of the chives.

Nutritional information:

3/4 cup makes one serving

- Calories-297
- Protein 11.4 grams
- Fat-26.6 grams
- Fiber-0.5 grams
- Carbs-3 grams

Tomato avocados

You will need 15 minutes for this

You will get 4 servings from this

You will need:

- 2 bacon slices
- A quarter teaspoon of garlic powder
- A single teaspoon of lime juice
- Half of a cup of halved grape tomatoes
- 2 avocados that are medium in size
- Half a cup of chopped romaine lettuce

What you will need:

1.   Get a skillet.
2.   Place your bacon inside the skillet while the pan is still cold.
3.   Cook bacon on low or medium-low heat. You want the edges to curl.
4.   Flip the bacon.
5.   Continue cooking until it becomes crispy and golden in color.
6.   This can take 5 minutes or longer.
7.   Drain on paper towels.
8.   Slice your avocados in half.
9.   Leave half of the halves alone but scoop the middle out of the other halves.
10.   Put it in a bowl.

11.   Mash the avocados that you put in the bowl and add in the rest of your ingredients besides the bacon.

12.   When the bacon has cooled, chop it up.

13.   Add to the bowl.

14.   Scoop the mixture in the bowl into all of the halves

Nutritional information:

One serving is half an avocado with filing

- Calories-189
- Fat-16 grams
- Fiber-7 grams
- Carbs-10 grams
- Protein-4 grams

Egg pie

You will need 40 minutes for this

You will get 6 servings from this

You will need:

- 2 slices of diced bacon
- A single spring of finely sliced onion
- 8 medium eggs
- 4.2 fluid ounces of full-fat milk
- 3 and a half ounces of shredded cheese

You will need to do the following:

1. Get a bowl.
2. Whisk your milk and eggs with a fork.
3. Add everything else to the bowl and stir gently.
4. Get a 20 by 8 baking dish and grease it and line it with baking paper.
5. Bake at 350 degrees for a half-hour.

Nutritional information:

- Calories-201
- Fat-17.7 grams
- Carbs-1.4 grams
- Protein-18 grams

Turkey Roll

You will need five minutes for this

You can get two servings out of this

You will need:

- A sliced avocado
- 2 ounces of lettuce
- 4 tablespoons of olive oil
- 3 ounces of cream cheese
- 6 ounces of turkey (use deli turkey)
- Salt and pepper for some flavor or taste if you like

What you will need to do:

1. Roll your turkey.
2. Arrange the vegetables around the turkey on a plate to make it look pleasing.
3. Arrange the cream cheese on the plate.
4. Drizzle olive oil over your vegetables and season with pepper and salt if need be.

Nutritional information:

- Calories-660
- Fat-60 grams
- Fiber-7 grams
- Protein-22 grams
- Carbs-7 grams

Roast beef rolls

You will need 5 minutes for this

You will get 2 servings from this

You will need:

- A single avocado
- A single scallion
- A half of a cup of mayo
- 5 ounces of cheese (use cheddar)
- Half a dozen radishes (six)
- 2 ounces of lettuce
- 2 tablespoons of olive oil
- 7 ounces of roast beef (use deli roast beef)
- A single tablespoon of mustard (use dijon)
- Salt and pepper for flavor

What you will need to do:

1. Roll the roast beef and set it on the plate, leaving room for the cheese and vegetables to go in between.
2. Put the sauces in the middle for dipping.
3. When you are ready to eat it, you can serve it with the lettuce and the olive oil over the top of the veggies for a great flavor.

Nutritional information:

- Calories-1071
- Fat-98 grams
- Fiber-8 grams
- Protein-38 grams
- Carbs-6 grams

Shrimp eggs

You will need 10 minutes to prepare

You will get 4 servings from this

What you need:

- Fresh dill
- A quarter cup of mayo
- A single teaspoon of tabasco
- A pinch of salt (use herbal salt)
- 4 eggs
- 8 cooked shrimp

What you will need:

1. Get a pot and begin boiling your eggs.
2. Boil the eggs for a minimum of eight minutes and a maximum of ten.
3. Remove the eggs from your pot.
4. Give them an ice bath for a few minutes.
5. Peel your eggs.
6. Split the eggs in half before scooping out the yolks.
7. Get yourself a bowl.
8. Mask the yolks in the bowl and add in your mayo, tabasco sauce, and salt.
9. Add the mixture to the eggs and place a shrimp on top.

Nutritional information:

- Calories-163
- Carbs-0.5 grams
- Protein-7 grams
- Fat-15 grams

Chapter 6: Snack Recipes

Chips

You only need five minutes to make this!

You will get four servings from this

What you need for the chip:

- A bag of pork rinds (take note that whatever bag you choose will change the nutrition information at the end of the recipe)
- Oil spray (make sure its avocado)

What you need for the coating:

- A single tablespoon of paprika
- ½ of a tablespoon of cayenne pepper for a little bit of a kick
- ½ of a tablespoon of onion powder
- ¼ of a cup of nutritional yeast
- ½ garlic powder

What you need to do:

1. Add the coating ingredients to a spice grinder and blend until everything becomes smooth.
2. Spray your pork rinds with oil as it will make the coating stick better.

3. Transfer the rinds to a plastic bag and pour the
   toppings in before you begin to shake it.

Nutritional information:

- Calories-97
- Fat-2.7 grams
- Carbs-2 grams
- Fiber- 1 gram
- Protein-14 grams

Pickle time!

This will only take you five minutes

You can get up to four servings from this

What you need:

- A single can of tuna (go for a version that is light flaked)
- ¼ of a cup of mayo (it needs to be sugar-free if you can get it and a light version)
- A single tablespoon of dill
- 5 or 6 pickles depending on what you need

What you need to do:

1. Cut your pickles in half so that they are lengthwise.
2. Seed your pickles.
3. Drain the tuna and then mix the dill, mayo, and tuna in a bowl before mixing.
4. Spoon the tuna mix onto the pickle.

Nutritional information:

A serving size here is based on if you used six pickles. Another note is that the nutritional information will change depending on what mayo you choose here.

- Calories-47.1
- Fiber-1.4 grams
- Protein 6.01 grams
- Carbs- 3.6 grams
- Fat-0.6

Hard-boiled eggs

You will need about 20 minutes to cook them and then time to cool them

You will be able to get twelve servings from this

What you need:

- A dozen eggs

What you need to do:

1. Get a pot that is big enough to hold the eggs.
2. Place six of the eggs in the pot.
3. Cover the eggs with cool water by an inch.
4. Cover your pan with a lid and bring your water to boiling.
5. Boil water in the pot for six minutes over medium-high heat
6. If you want them firmer, let them stay in the pot a little longer.
7. Repeat for the other six.

This is perfect for taking on the go and makes a quick protein-packed snack.

Nutritional information:

This is based upon two eggs.

- Calories-156
- Carbs-1 gram
- Fiber-o grams
- Fat-10.6 grams
- Protein-12.6 grams

Zingy crackers

You will need 25 minutes for this

You will get 16 pieces

You will need:

- A single pound cheddar cheese (sliced)
- 4 sliced jalapeno peppers (use sliced)

What you will need to do:

1. Heat oven to 425 and then line your baking sheet with parchment
2. Cut your cheese slices. They need to be 11/2 inch squares.
3. Arrange them on the baking sheet with at least an inch between them and then place a slice of jalapeno on top.
4. You will then place them in the oven and bake for a dozen minutes (12) .
5. You will know they are done when they are firm and light brown.
6. Remove and let them cool.
7. If stored in an airtight container, they will last two days.

Nutritional information:

- Calories-106
- Protein-7 grams
- Carbs-1 gram
- Fiber-0.3 grams
- Fat-9 grams

Pinwheel Delight

You will need ten minutes for this

You will get 20 pieces from this

What you need:

- A single block of cream cheese (8 ounces)
- 10 slices of salami (genoa) and pepperoni
- 4 tablespoons of pickles (make sure they are finely diced)

What you need to do:

1. Have your cream cheese brought to room temperature.
2. Whip the cream cheese until it becomes fluffy.
3. Spread your cream cheese in a rectangle that is a quarter-inch thick. Do this on a large piece of plastic wrap.
4. Place your pickles over cream cheese
5. Place the salami over the cream cheese in layers that are overlapping so that each cream cheese layer is covered.
6. Place another layer of wrap over the layer of salami and press down. Be gentle.
7. Flip your whole rectangle over so that the bottom cream cheese layer is now facing the top instead.
8. Peel back your plastic wrap off very carefully from the top cream cheese layer.

9. You should begin rolling this into a log shape, slowly removing the bottom layer of your plastic wrap as you go along.
10. Place the pinwheel in a tight plastic wrap.
11. Place in the fridge overnight or if you can't wait at least four hours.
12. Slice however thick you want it.

Nutritional information:

- Calories- 47
- Fat-4.2 grams
- Protein-1 gram
- Carbs-0.8 grams

This is based on a single pinwheel

Zesty olives

You will need 10 minutes for this recipe

You will get up to 6 servings out of this maximum and 4 at a minimum

What you need:

- 1/4 of a cup of oil (make sure that it is extra virgin olive oil)
- 1/4 of a teaspoon of pepper flakes (red and crushed)
- A single thinly sliced garlic clove
- A single tablespoon of lemon juice
- A single strip of zest from a lemon
- A single cup of olives (make sure that they are castelvetrano)
- 2 sprigs of thyme (make sure it's fresh)
- A single tablespoon of orange juice
- A single strip of zest from an orange

What you need to do:

1. Get a saucepan.
2. Heat your oil over a heat that is medium-high.
3. Add zest, thyme, garlic, and zest in and cook it.
4. Be sure that you stir occasionally.
5. Cook for a few minutes, and you will notice that the garlic is golden.
6. You will then need to stir in the olives and cook them as well.

7. Stir them as they cook but only cook for two minutes. You want them to be warmed.
8. Turn off your heat.
9. Stir in your juice.
10. Place in a dish.

Nutritional information:

- Calories-180
- Fat- 20 grams
- Carbs- 2 grams

Deviled Eggs Keto Style!

This takes 10 minutes
You can get 20 deviled eggs here

What you need:

- 10 eggs (hardboiled of course)
- 10 large eggs, hardboiled
- A single avocado (make sure it is ripe)
- A single lemon (you will need to juice this)
- A single tablespoon of mustard (use Dijon)
- Paprika (use smoked)

What you need to do:

1. Slice your eggs in half and take out the yolks.
2. Combine your yolks, avocado, and lemon juice in a bowl and stir thoroughly.
3. Spoon the mixture into the egg halves.
4. Sprinkle the top with paprika.

Nutritional information:

- Calories-50
- Fat-4 grams
- Fiber-1 gram
- Protein- 3 grams
- Carbs- 1 gram

Cucumber time

You will need 5 minutes for this

You will get one serving from this

What you will need:

- A single cup of cucumbers (make sure they are sliced)
- 10 olived (kalamata olives. Use large ones)

What you need to do:

1. Mix them together in a bowl, and there you go!

Nutritional information:

- Calories-71
- Fiber-2.3 grams
- Carbs-5 grams
- Fat-4.8 grams
- Protein-1.29 grams

Nutty Yogurt

This will take 5 minutes

It will give you one serving

What you need:

- 2 ounces of yogurt (use whole milk greek yogurt)
- 1/2 of a teaspoon of cinnamon
- 1 tablespoon of walnuts (chopped)

What you need to do:

1. Place the yogurt in a dish.
2. Add the walnuts.
3. Add the cinnamon.

Nutritional information:

- Calories-160
- Fiber-0.5 grams
- Fat-12.5 grams
- Protein-8 grams
- Carbs-6 grams

Let's Get Crabby!

You will need 10 minutes for this

You can get 4 servings from this

What you need:

- A single avocado (make sure that it is ripe)
- 3 tablespoons of juice from a lemon.
- 2 tablespoons of chives (chopped)
- 1/2 of a pound of crab meat (lump)
- 1 teaspoon of mustard (use dijon)

What you need to do:

1. Put your avocados.
2. Peel them next.
3. Cut into chunks a half-inch thick.
4. Place them in a bowl.
5. Add a tablespoon of your juice.
6. In a separate bowl, add your other ingredients except the meat and whisk it together.
7. Add the meat and toss the ingredients.
8. Do the same for the last three servings.

Nutritional information:

- Calories-150
- Fat-8 grams
- Protein-15 grams
- Carbs-5 grams
- Fiber-3 grams

Cream And Berries

You will need 5 minutes to prepare this

You will get one serving from this

What you need:

- A quarter of a cup of berries (raspberries are best)
- A single cup of whipping cream

What you need to do:

1. Place the whipping cream on the bottom of your bowl.
2. Place your berries on top.

Nutritional information:

- Calories-230
- Fat-21.5 grams
- Protein-2 grams
- Fiber- 4 grams
- Carbs-5.1 grams

Let's go boating

You will need 5 minutes for this

You will get one serving out of this

What you need:

- A single celery stalk
- 2 tablespoons of peanut butter
- Chia seeds for the top if you desire to do so (it will give you a bit of omega-3s)

What you will need to do:

1. Cut the stalk into pieces after making sure that it is clean.
2. Place the peanut butter on top.
3. If you have chosen to use chia seeds, add them as well.

Nutritional information:

- Calories-225
- Fat-18.3 grams
- Fiber-4.6 grams
- Protein-9.3 grams
- Carbs-9.8 grams

Guacamole break

You will need five minutes for this

You will get a single serving from this

What you need:

- Half a cup of guacamole
- Half of a cucumber

What you need to do:

1. Cut the cucumber into slices after cleaning it.
2. Serve with the guacamole.

Nutritional information:

- Calories- 233
- Fat-19.9 grams
- Fiber-7.7 grams
- Carbs-14.9 grams
- Protein-3.2 grams

Creamy Dream

You will need five minutes for this

You will get one serving with this

What you need:

- 2 tablespoons almond butter (go with creamy it will mix better)
- A single teaspoon of flax seeds
- 2 teaspoons of pumpkin seeds
- A single teaspoon of sunflower seeds
- A single teaspoon of chia seeds

What you need to do:

1. Get a bowl.
2. Mix all the ingredients together.

The protein that you will get along with the fiber and fat should work to keep you full for longer.

Nutritional information:

- Calories-262
- Fat-21 grams
- Carbs-11.6 grams
- Protein-11 grams
- Fiber-7.8 grams

Creamy boat

You will need five minutes for this

You will get 2 servings from this

What you will need:

- 2 stalks of celery
- 2 tablespoons of cream cheese

What you need to do:

1. Clean the celery and cut it into pieces.
2. Place the pieces on a plate before adding cream cheese to them.
3. Repeat this process if necessary.

Nutritional information:

- Calories-113
- Fat-10.1 grams
- Fiber-1.3 grams
- Carbs-4 grams
- Protein-2.3 grams

Tomato Attack!

You will need 5 minutes for this

You will get one serving from this

What you need:

- 2 tablespoons of seeds (go with pumpkin on this one)
- Half a cup of cottage cheese (make sure it's full fat)
- A single teaspoon of olive oil
- 5 cherry tomato halves

What you need to do:

1. Place the halves on a plate in any formation, but a flower or a pattern that will leave the middle open for the cottage cheese is best.
2. The pumpkin seeds will make a great topping for the cottage cheese.

If you choose to add other vegetables like bell peppers, it will change the nutritional value, so be aware of this.

Nutritional information:

- Calories-201
- fat- 10.9 grams
- Protein-14.2 grams
- Fiber-2.5 grams
- Carbs-7.9 grams

Kabobs

You will need 5 minutes for this

You will get one serving out of this

What you need:

- A single ounce of salami (try to get a high quality if you can such as from a deli)
- A single ounce of cheese (your choice but you can have fun mixing and matching)

What you need to do:

1. Get a kabob stick and begin placing the cheese and meat upon it.
2. When you done, it's ready to be enjoyed.

Nutritional information:

- Calories-215
- Fat-16.5 grams
- Protein-14.8 grams
- Carbs-0.6 grams

Get your grapefruit on

You need 5 minutes for this

You will get one serving out of this

It's important to note here that grapefruit is only allowed on the keto diet in small doses.

What you need:

- ¼ of a grapefruit (use segments)
- ½ of a cup of cottage cheese

What you need to do to:

1. Get a bowl.
2. Place the cottage cheese at the bottom.
3. Place the grapefruit on the top.

Nutritional information:

- Calories-136
- Protein-12.5 grams
- Carbs-11.6 grams
- Fat-5.1 grams
- fiber- 1 grams

Veggie sandwich

You will need 5 minutes for this

You will get one serving

What you need:

- A single red pepper
- 2 slices of deli ham

If you need more fat in your snack, then you can add some avocado for the needed nutrition. Just note that it will change your nutritional information below.

You can also add more vegetables if you want to as well.

What you need to do:

Cut your pepper in half and take the seeds out. Place one half on a plate then stick the meat inside. Place the other half of the pepper over the top.

Nutritional information:

- Calories-101
- Protein011.2 grams
- Carbs-9.2 grams
- Fiber-2.5 grams
- Fat-2.9 grams

Cheese plate

You need five minutes for this

You will get one serving from this

What you need:

- ½ of a cup of cherry tomatoes
- An ounce of brie (this is a great cheese to use because it has no carbs)

What you need to do:

1. Place your tomatoes and cheese on a plate. If you like, you can get creative with how you do this. It looks pretty if you place the tomatoes in flower.

Nutritional information:

- Calories-133
- Fat-11.2 grams
- Carbs-2.9 grams
- Protein-4.7 grams
- Fiber-0.9 grams

Mini salad

You will need 10 minutes for this

You will get one serving from this

What you need:

- One egg (large and hard-boiled)
- ½ of a teaspoon of mustard
- A single tablespoon of mayo

What you need to do:

1. Peel the egg.
2. Mash it up well in a bowl.
3. Combine the mayo and mustard with the mashed egg.

Nutritional information

- Calorie-175
- Carbs-0.5 grams
- Protein-6.5 grams
- Fat-15 grams

Pickle wrap

You will need ten minutes for this recipe

You will get a single serving

What you need:

- A dill pill (use a large one)
- One ounce of sliced cheese
- One ounce of deli meat (sliced)

Depending on what you choose this will alter the numbers

What you need to do:

1. This is where you can get creative. You can either wrap the entire pickle with the meat and cheese, or you can cut it into slices or halves and wrap it. However, you want it to work for you.

Nutritional information:

- Calories-260
- Carbs-3 grams
- Fiber-1.5 grams
- Protein-6 grams
- Fat-9.5 grams

Meatless wraps

You will need 5 minutes for this recipe

You will get one serving from this

What you will need:

- A large collard green leaf (make sure it has no stem)
- An ounce of cheddar cheese (it will need to be sliced)
- A teaspoon of mustard (use dijon)
- A teaspoon of mayo

What you need to do:

1. Take the green leaf and spread the condiments on it before adding the cheese.
2. Then roll it like a wrap.

Nutritional information:

- Calories-162
- Fat-13.4 grams
- Carbs-1.3 grams
- Fiber-1.5 grams
- Protein-8.2 grams

Lettuce cup

You will need five minutes for this

You will get one serving

What you need to have:

- 2 ounces of tuna (canned)
- 2 tablespoons of mayo
- A lettuce leaf

What you need to do:

1. Lay the lettuce leaf flat.
2. Spread the mayo on the leaf.
3. Spread the tuna over the top.
4. Fold the lettuce into a cup shape.

Nutritional information:

- Calories-261
- Fat-22.3 grams
- Protein-13.6 grams
- Carbs-0.1 grams

Let's get Cheesy!

You will need 5 minutes for this

You will get one serving from this

What you will need:

- A quarter of a cup of cheese (use shredded and cheddar)
- 2 tablespoons of sunflower seeds
- A single can of tuna
- 2 tablespoons of mayo

What you need to do:

1. Grab a bowl.
2. Mix everything but the cheese together.
3. Add in your cheese and either leave it on the top or mix it in well as well to combine it.

Nutritional information:

- Calories-265
- Fat-21 grams
- Fiber-1 gram
- Carbs-2 grams
- Protein-17 grams

Cocoa Balls

You will need 5 minutes to make this recipe with additional time for cooling

You will get one serving from this

What you need:

- A single tablespoon of peanut butter (make sure it's natural and smooth)
- A sprinkle of cocoa powder (make sure it's unsweetened)

What you need to do:

1. Roll your peanut butter in your hands to form a ball.
2. When you have the right feel, sprinkle the ball with the powder
3. Place in a bowl and let it chill for an hour in the fridge.

Nutritional information:

- Calories-101
- Fat-8.3 grams
- Fiber-2.5 grams
- Protein-4.5 grams
- Carbs-5 grams

Veggie Sushi

You will need 20 minutes for this recipe

You will get 4 servings from this

What you need:

- 2 carrots (you need small ones, and they need to be sliced thinly)
- A quarter of an avocado (sliced thinly)
- 2 cucumbers (use medium ones and halve them)
- ½ of a bell pepper (yellow and thinly sliced)
- ½ of a bell pepper (red and thinly sliced)

If you choose to dip them, what you will need for the dip is as follows:

- A single teaspoon of soy sauce
- A single tablespoon of sriracha (for a kick in flavor)
- ⅓ of a cup of mayo

What you will need to do:

1. Use a spoon to remove the center of the cucumbers. You want them hollow.
2. Put your avocado in the center and then slide your other veggies inside that hole so that the hole is full of veggies.

3. In a small dish, make the sauce to dip the sushi in.
4. Slice the cucumber into pieces and place on a plate with the sauce.

Nutritional information:

- Calories-190
- Protein- 1 gram
- Carbs-9 grams
- Fiber-3 grams
- Fat-16 grams

Cheese bites

You will need about 20 minutes for this

You will get 4 servings for this

What you will need:

- 8 ounces of cheddar cheese (make sure that it's shredded)
- ½ teaspoon of paprika (powder)

What you will need to do:

1. Preheat your oven to 400 degrees
2. Add your cheese into a small little heaps on your baking sheet after lining it with parchment paper.
3. Make sure to leave room between each heap and that they are not touching.
4. Sprinkle your paprika over the heaps.
5. Bake for a minimum of eight minutes and a maximum of ten minutes.
6. Pay close attention that you don't burn the cheese.
7. Let them cool before you eat them.

Nutritional information:

- Calories-231
- Protein-13 grams
- Carbs-3 grams
- Fat-19 grams

Lettuce for your thoughts?

You will need five minutes for this

You will get a single serving out of this

What you will need:

- A single cherry tomato
- ½ of an ounce of butter
- A single ounce of cheese of your liking. For this recipe, we are using edam.
- 2 ounces of romaine lettuce
- ½ of an avocado

What you will need to do:

1. Make sure that you clean the lettuce thoroughly and then use the lettuce as a boat to hold the rest of the ingredients.
2. Spread butter over the lettuce, and then slice your ingredients before placing them on the top.

A fun idea is that you can put just about any vegetable or even tuna on top of the lettuce, and you will have a nutritious meal.

Nutritional information:

- Calories-374
- Protein-10 grams
- Fat-34 grams
- Carbs- 4 grams
- Fiber-8 grams

Chocolate cake

You will only need minutes for this

You will get one serving of cake from this

What you need:

- A single tablespoon of chocolate chips (use sugar-free ones)
- 2 tablespoons of melted butter
- A single tablespoon of coconut flour
- A single tablespoon of cocoa powder
- An egg that has been beaten
- ⅛ of a teaspoon of vanilla extract
- ½ a teaspoon of baking powder
- 2 tablespoons of erythritol (swerve is what we're using here)
- 2 tablespoons of almond flour
- A single pinch of salt

What you need to do:

1. Get yourself a large coffee mug.
2. Add the egg, vanilla, and egg.
3. Mix it well.
4. Add in your dry ingredients and mix it well as you did the wet ingredients.
5. Microwave on high for a minute.
6.

If you overcook it, your cake will be dry, and it won't taste right.

Nutritional information:

- Calories-397
- Fat-37 grams
- Fiber-6 grams
- Protein-12 grams
- Carbs-10 grams

Conclusion

The ketogenic diet is one that has many important aspects and information that you need to know as someone who wants to try this diet. It is important to remember the warning that we have given you at the beginning of the book that this is not a diet that is safe and that doctors recommend you don't try it, or if you are going to attempt it remember that you shouldn't do so for longer than six months and even then never without the constant supervision of a doctor or at the very least a doctor knowing that your doing this and you following their guidelines and words exactly so that they can make sure that you are safe.

The ketogenic diet is a diet that believes that by minimizing your carbs, you will while maximizing the good fat in your system and making sure that you're getting the protein you need, that you will be happier and healthier. In this book we give you the information to know what this diet is all about as well as describing the different types and areas that this diet will offer. Most people assume that there is only one way to do this and while there is one thing that the additional options share, there are actually four different options you can choose from. Each one has it's unique benefits, and you should know about each type to learn what would be best for your body, which is why we have described them in the book for you to have the best information possible when you begin this diet for yourself.

Another big thing about this diet is that many people don't understand the importance of exercise with this diet. The best way to become healthier is to do three things for yourself. Get the right amount of sleep, eat healthily, and make sure that you get the proper amount of exercise as well for your body to work at an optimum level. As such we explain the exercises that are the best to go with your diet to make sure that you are getting the most out of it.

For women who are on the go and have a busy lifestyle, we have provided recipes for a thirty-day meal plan so that you can make food quickly and have a great meal for your lifestyle. They also have enough servings for you to have leftovers so that you don't have to worry about preparing in the morning. Instead, you can simply pack it up and take it with you wherever you go. This works out so much easier for so many people because they don't have to cook in the morning, and it saves a busy person a lot of time.

We also provide helpful ideas on how you can use these recipes for meals to make sure that you see how the numbers will affect you and make an impact on your day. A great example that we have explained is if you have a big breakfast that is full of the protein you need, for example, thirty grams, you've got to take note of this and be aware because if you eat too much for your dinner or another meal, you will throw your numbers out of where they are supposed to be. For those that have more time on their hands, we offer a thirty-day meal plan for you as well with all-new recipes to enjoy and tips and tricks for making them work for you in the best way.

With all of this information at your fingertips, you will be able to enjoy this diet and use it to your advantage. Another benefit that we offer? We explain routines that you can do for yourself to make this diet last longer for you and to benefit your body better as a result. Routines are very important and can be a big help to your body but also your spirit and your mind. This will help you utilize the diet better, and you will be able to improve with it as well as have it become easier for you to handle.

As many people are using this diet to their benefit, knowing your food is one of the biggest parts of this, and it becomes easier once you begin to use this in your daily life. One of the best things you can do is pay attention to the food that your eating and how it affects your body and mind. You will notice that this diet has the ability to make you sick, which isn't a good thing and it's one of the things the doctors warn against. For this reason it's very important to pay attention to what your eating and how your feeling at the same time. Another warning that we have said you need to pay attention to is that you will need to make sure that your ketogenic 'flu' isn't the result of something more serious. As people are being told that this is normal, this book has brought you the knowledge you need to be able to tell you why it's not.

This book has given you all the information you need to do this diet properly and to do it well. It's important to understand what you're getting into when you go into this diet, and this book will give you valuable information that you can use to your benefit and so you can avoid the problems that can come with this diet. You want to stay healthy and make sure that your body is able to do what it needs to. As with anything, we have put a strong emphasis on the fact that if anything feels wrong or unnatural you will need to see a doctor to make sure that you are safe and that your body can handle this diet. Use the knowledge in this book to have amazing recipes and learn how to prepare amazing meals for yourself.

www.ingramcontent.com/pod-product-compliance
Lightning Source LLC
Chambersburg PA
CBHW070656250726
48662CB00001B/142